*Routledge Revivals*

---

# The Story of Modern Preventive Medicine

First published in 1929, this book is a continuation of Arthur Newsholme's *Evolution of Preventive Medicine*, published in 1927, which was concerned with the possibilities in the progress of prevention of disease, up to the middle of the nineteenth century. The current volume focuses on the modern period and looks at the work of Louis Pasteur in particular. It provides a complete overview of the subject of preventive medicine at the time and should be used as the basis for more detailed study. The book will be useful to those in medical circles, as well as historians interested in medicine.

# The Story of Modern Preventive Medicine

## Being a Continuation of the Evolution of Preventive Medicine

Sir Arthur Newsholme

Routledge
Taylor & Francis Group
Routledge Revivals

First published in 1929
by The Williams and Wilkins Company

This edition first published in 2015 by Routledge
4 Park Square, Milton Park, Abingdon, Oxon OX14 4RN
605 Third Avenue, New York, NY 10017

*Routledge is an imprint of the Taylor & Francis Group, an informa business*



A Library of Congress record exists under LC control number: 29004701

ISBN 13: 978-1-138-90801-7 (hbk)
ISBN 13: 978-1-315-69317-0 (ebk)

# THE STORY OF MODERN PREVENTIVE MEDICINE

*BEING A CONTINUATION OF THE EVOLUTION OF PREVENTIVE MEDICINE, 1927*

*By*

SIR ARTHUR NEWSHOLME, K.C.B., M.D., F.R.C.P.

*Formerly Principal Medical Officer of the Local Government Board of England, and Lecturer on Public Health Administration, School of Hygiene and Public Health, The Johns Hopkins University*

*Made in United States of America*

Published January, 1929

Composed and Printed at the
WAVERLY PRESS
for
The Williams & Wilkins Company
Baltimore, Md., U. S. A.

# PREFACE

As stated in the title-page, this volume is a continuation of "Evolution of Preventive Medicine," published in 1927, which was concerned with the progress in possibilities of prevention of disease up to the middle of the nineteenth century. In the present volume this sketch is continued through the modern period ushered in by Louis Pasteur's work.

No strict line of demarcation between the earlier and the later period can, however, be drawn; and in dealing, for instance, with two diseases of such world-wide importance as tuberculosis and syphilis it has been necessary to outline both the earlier and the later periods of growth of possibilities of prevention of disease. Similar remarks apply to some other diseases, and especially to malaria and yellow fever. But in the main the present volume deals with the scientific, while the earlier volume was concerned chiefly with the pre-scientific period of disease prevention.

The same limitations as were prescribed for the earlier volume hold good for the Story in the present volume. It is elementary and in outline only, and is to be regarded as preliminary to more detailed study of the work of individual investigators, of individual diseases, and of special branches of research. Restrictions of space, furthermore, have necessarily implied that some branches of prevention and the work of some investigators on which it would be pleasant to write, have been passed by.

I cannot hope that in the crowded record of the following pages I have entirely avoided inaccuracies, though every care has been taken. Perhaps more serious is the omission of the names of living investigators whose work should have received adequate mention. These omissions and possible errors will not be serious, if the reading of my preliminary sketch stimulates students and social and medical workers to more detailed study of the progress in disease prevention and health improvement already secured and of the great possibilities for the future.

The writing of this sketch, and the associated review of the investigations on which has been based the work in which I have been engaged during four and a half decades, has at least given me a pleasant task; while this long experience of public health administration—which consists in application of our knowledge of preventive medicine—should have enabled me to present the Story of the Growth of Knowledge of the principles of preventive medicine not altogether out of perspective.

ARTHUR NEWSHOLME

*The Athenæum*
*Pall Mall, London*
*July, 1928*

# CONTENTS

## PART I. THE PREVENTION OF SPECIFIC DISEASES

### CHAPTER I

INTRODUCTORY CONSIDERATIONS........................ 3
Evidences of improved vitality.—Quality and quantity of life.—Chief causes of death.—Age distribution of deaths—Definition of premature death.

### CHAPTER II

CAUSATION OF DISEASE.............................. 12
Specificity.—Experimental and experiential investigation.—Pathological and clinical investigation.—Laennec and Bretonneau.—"Physiological Medicine." —Villemin and Virchow.—Etiological nosography.— —Specific therapeutics.—Terrain and microbe.

### CHAPTER III

THE EARLIER WORK OF PASTEUR AND HIS PREDECESSORS. 23
Spontaneous generation.—Omne vivum ex ovo.

### CHAPTER IV

THE FIRST AND GREATEST TRIUMPH IN APPLICATION OF GERM THEORY.................................. 29
Pyogenic diseases.—Air of hospitals?—Joseph Lister. —Anaesthetics and Lister's work.—Stages in development of antisepticism (including asepticism).

CHAPTER V

EARLIER DISCOVERIES IN BACTERIOLOGY.............. 37
Anthrax. Specificity of bacteria?—Technique of discoveries.—Pasteur and Koch.—Earlier work on anthrax.—Koch's demonstration.—Pasteur's work on anthrax.

CHAPTER VI

EARLIER ATTEMPTS AT SPECIFIC PROPHYLAXIS.......... 46
Explanation of immunity.—Fowl cholera attenuation.—A new method of vaccination.—Greenfield's work.—Attenuation of virulence of anthrax bacilli.—Experiments on sheep and cattle.

CHAPTER VII

THE PREVENTION OF RABIES......................... 52
Experimentation with an unknown virus. Pasteur's work on rabbits.—Application to man.—Britain's experimental eradication of rabies.

CHAPTER VIII

THE PREVENTION OF DIPHTHERIA...................... 60
Localisation of specific bacilli.—Work of Roux and Behring.—Serum of immunes curative.—Statistical evidence.—Production of active immunisation.—Diagnosis of susceptibility by cutaneous reaction.

CHAPTER IX

BACTERIOLOGY IN RELATION TO IMMUNITY AND TO DIAGNOSIS......................................... 72
Small pox.—Phagocytosis.—Pfeiffer's phenomenon.—Serum diagnosis.—Protective vaccination for tetanus, cholera, typhoid fever, diphtheria, scarlet fever.—Ehrlich's work.

## CHAPTER X

The Prevention of Cholera........................ 81
Pandemicity.—Relation to sanitation.—Pettenkofer's localist hypothesis.—Hamburg epidemic.

## CHAPTER XI

The Prevention of Enteric or Typhoid Fever....... 88
The Eberth bacillus.—Relation to water supplies.—Illustrations.—Methods of water purification.—Shell fish and carriers in relation to typhoid.—Sanitary defects.

## CHAPTER XII

The Prevention of Undulant (Malta or Mediterranean) Fever.................................. 106
Discovery of *M. melitensis* and agglutinins.—Presence in goat's milk.—A single vehicle of infection?

## CHAPTER XIII

The Prevention of Louse-Borne Diseases.......... 111
Relapsing fever.—Typhus fever.—Nicolle's work.—A modified type of typhus.—Importation a necessary condition of prevalence.—Trench fever.

## CHAPTER XIV

Hookworm Disease (Ankylostomiasis)............... 120
Characteristics.—Loos's discovery of method of infection. Conditions of prevalence.—Miner's anaemia.—Closet provision.—Bare feet.—Therapeutic prevention.

## CHAPTER XV

The Prevention of Plague........................ 126
Pandemicity.—*Bacillus pestis*.—Spread by rat fleas.—Simond's views.—Investigation by Plague Commission.—Experimental proof of methods of transmission.

CHAPTER XVI

Filariasis and Texas Fever........................ 134
House fly and disease.—Manson's investigation of filaria.—Proof of transmission by mosquito.—Texas fever and ticks.—Theobald Smith's work.

CHAPTER XVII

The Prevention of Malaria........................ 143
History of malaria.—Laveran, Ross, Golgi, MacCallum, Grassi.—Manson's foresight.—Experimental proof in Britain.

CHAPTER XVIII

The Prevention of Yellow Fever.................. 154
Pandemicity.—Carter's epidemiological work.—Work of Walter Reed and colleagues.—Previous work and surmises.—Gorgas' practical application in Cuba and Panama.

CHAPTER XIX

The Prevention of Venereal Diseases............ 164
Magnitude of mischief.—History of syphilis.—Experimental production of syphilis.—Prophylaxis by calomel.—Laboratory diagnosis.—Prevention and cure by 606.—Specific cure.

CHAPTER XX

The Prevention of Tuberculosis.................. 174
History of the disease.—Villemin's pioneer work.—Koch's and the tubercle bacillus.—Influence of foul air, of occupation, of poverty.—Origin from cow's milk.—Influence of dosage of infection.—Tuberculisation.—Immunisation.—Therapeutic treatment and prevention.

## PART II. SOME PHYSICAL AND SOCIAL CONDITIONS OF HEALTH

### CHAPTER XXI

Air and Ventilation .................................. 195
Evils of expired air.—Moving and still air.—Flügge and Haldane.—Thermal not chemical problem.—Dust in air.—Effluvia of drains and sewers.—Bacterial content of air.—Droplet and dust infection in tuberculosis, etc.

### CHAPTER XXII

Fog, Smoke, Sunlight.................................. 211
Soot in air.—Relation of fog to smoke.—Experimental investigation of sunlight and health.—Effect of ultraviolet rays. Helio-therapy.

### CHAPTER XXIII

Housing and Occupation.............................. 217
Improved housing.—Inimical influences of urbanisation.—Occupational history.—Ramazzini and Thackrah.—Dust and phthisis.—Phosphorus and lead poisoning.—Anthrax.—Cancer and occupation.—Industrial fatigue.

## PART III. SOME PHYSIOLOGICAL CONDITIONS OF HEALTH

### CHAPTER XXIV

The Prevention of Goitre and Cretinism... ........ 233
History of discovery of thyroid functions.—Iodine metabolism.

CHAPTER XXV

Excess and Deficiencies of Food .................. 238
Gluttony.—Gout.—Factors in defective nutrition.—Borderland conditions.—Disease of defect.—Bread and milk.

CHAPTER XXVI

Hormones and Vitamins .................. 246
Indebtedness to chemistry.—Fermentation.—Hormones.—Food hormones.—Hopkins' and other investigations. — Vitamins. — Ergosterol. — Irradiation of foods.—Effect of cooking on vitamins.

CHAPTER XXVII

The Prevention of Rickets .................. 257
Results of rickets.—Experimental evidence on causation. Irradiation by ultra-violet rays.—Cod liver oil and sunlight.—Ergosterol.

CHAPTER XXVIII

The Prevention of Scurvy, Beri-Beri and Xerophthalmia .................. 267
Scurvy.—Experimental voyages.—Animal experimentation. — Beri-beri. — Eijkman's epidemiological work.—Funk's experimental work.—Keratomalacia —Occurrence in war.—Pellagra.

CHAPTER XXIX

The Prevention of the Alcoholic Evil .................. 277
International experience as to the evil.—Crime, disease, accidents, industrial inefficiency.—Occupational alcoholism.—Physiological effect of small doses.

Index .................. 289

# PART I

# THE PREVENTION OF SPECIFIC DISEASES

# CHAPTER I

## Introductory Considerations

In my previous volume *The Evolution of Preventive Medicine*, 1927, an elementary sketch was given of the growth of the idea of prevention of disease, and of the limited application which this idea has received in the treatment of disease throughout the ages. This sketch showed the slow growth of knowledge, the too slow defeat of doctrine by scientifically ascertained fact, the gradual weeding out of error from truth, and the fundamental discoveries in physiology, and to a limited extent in pathology, which have made possible further progress in preventive medicine.

My panoramic sketch—excepting only a bare enumeration of more recent progress in Chapter XXIII of the above work—stopped short at the time when the germ theory of disease became a scientifically acceptable doctrine. In this volume is attempted a similar elementary sketch of the History of Preventive Medicine in the years which have elapsed since the genius of Pasteur inaugurated the scientific study of communicable diseases, and made possible the preventive measures which ensued from that study.

Happily progress during the last seventy years has not been limited to the elucidation of the causes of diseases which are transmissible from man to man or from animals to man. There has occurred also a vast addition to our knowledge of physics, of chemistry, and of physiology as bearing on health, especially in regard to food and sunlight. In the final chapters which follow, these aspects of preventive medicine are briefly considered. On both the physiological and pathological side of preventive medicine, selection of available material is inevitable; and many advances in potential or actual prevention of disease are necessarily left to be studied in more detailed treatises, general and special.

In the remainder of this chapter we may indicate in brief outline some of the evidences of progress in preventive medicine already attained.

The test commonly employed to show improvement in vitality is to measure the average duration of life; and a few figures as to this may be given. Fuller information is contained in my *Elements of Vital Statistics in their Bearing on Social and Public Health Problems*, 1923. Length of days, however, is not the only object in preventive medicine. Another view is given in the statement in the Wisdom of Solomon (Apocrypha): "Honorable age is not that which standeth in length of time, nor is measured in number of years. He being made perfect in a short time fulfilled a long time."

Quality of life as well as quantity enters into consideration, and the attainment of a lower average standard of health and efficiency in a longer life may not be a worthy end. If mere material advance is the "target of our ambition," it forms a very inadequate justification for a public health campaign. Preventive medicine aims at improved quality of life in its physical, intellectual and moral aspects; and for the mass of mankind there has been vast improvement, at least, in the first two of these, as shown by physical health and in recreational and aesthetic life. With our increasing knowledge of the evolution of mind and of the possibilities of its training and cultivation, the scope of preventive medicine will ere long be increased, and "social diseases" may be diminished in volume to an extent the feasibilty of which as yet is very imperfectly realized.

The saving of life already secured, and especially of child life, has not resulted in a lower average standard of health for the increased number of survivors. Evidence of this is given in *Vital Statistics* (page 358). There is, for instance, a considerable volume of evidence that in fairly prosperous countries the average height and weight of children is improving.

The available evidence as to duration of life may be considered physiologically or statistically.

Life is defined sometimes as that which resists death; and experiments on lowly organisms confirm Dr. J. Loeb's statement that "death is not inherent in the individual cell, but is only the fate of more complicated organisms in which the different types of cells or tissues are dependent upon each other."

Body tissues have been cultivated outside the body just as have bacteria, and given suitable conditions fragments of the tissues of a chicken have been kept alive in plasma or a saline solution on a glass slide and have continued to grow and reproduce their cells for as long as twelve years, a period much longer than that of the natural life of a fowl. This proves, as Starling states, that "mortality is but an accident of the complexity of our living machine and not a necessary quality and fate of the tissues of which the body is composed."

In man, however, in whom many tissues and organs are necessary for continued life, the duration of life is limited by the integrity of each essential part and it can only be increased by search for and removâl of the enemies of this integrity.

In figure 1 are indicated the relative incidence of some of the heaviest causes of death, as illustrated by experience in the United States. It will be noted that cardiac diseases head the list; but it must be remembered that death certificates with this heading merely state the final condition in a sequence of morbid conditions of multiform origin; and that the real cause of death under the heading "heart disease" has been damaging rheumatic or other infection, especially in early life, syphilis in early adult life, or some other condition to which in the interest of preventive medicine attention is required more than to the consequential heart disease.

The other items do not call for special comment in this chapter, but it should be noted that if we include—as we should—bronchitis, pneumonia and influenza as of infectious origin, and even if we assume—contrary to the facts—that heart diseases, renal diseases, and diseases of early infancy are not also largely if not chiefly of infectious origin, nearly half of the deaths included in the diagram are due to infection from without. From a wider review of all

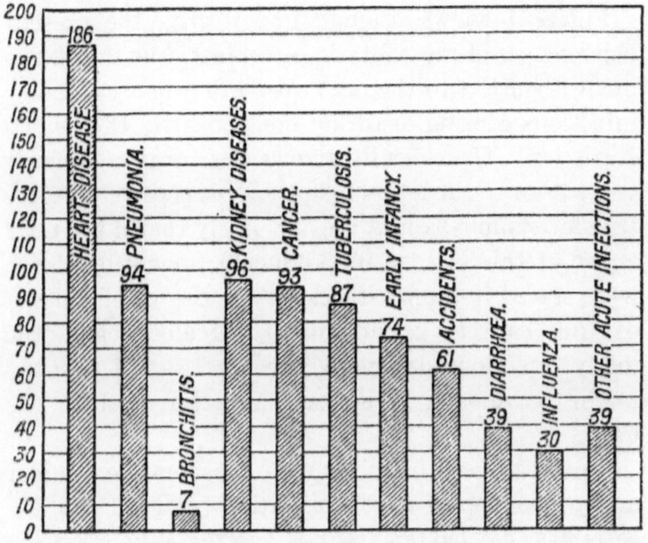


Fig. 1

causes of death it is no exaggeration to state that at least half of the practice of preventive medicine must continue to be concerned with the prevention of infection and the avoidance of circumstances favoring infection.

No line of demarcation can, however, be drawn,

and none should be attempted. Cause and consequence act and react: physiological and social circumstances favoring good health strengthen the defences against infection; while diminution of infection renders these circumstances much more favorable than otherwise they would be.

Figure 1 shows, though imperfectly, the present chief causes of mortality in our midst; but this statement is subject to the reservation that many primary infections causing death do not appear in the official statistics. Their deadly arrows were projected many years prior to the lethal result. This is pre-eminently true for syphilis; and it appears likely that if the total effect of this disease in producing premature death were stated it would stand among the chief thieves of life—cancer, pneumonia, tuberculosis, and the many infections damaging the heart,—and possibly might be almost, if not actually, foremost in the list.

As will be seen in subsequent chapters the number and proportion of deaths resulting from various diseases has changed remarkably; and these changes have had the general effect of increasing the average duration of life for each child at birth by ten to fifteen years in different communities. (See chapter XXII, *Vital Statistics*.)

The decrease in the risk of death at each period of life can also be shown by the death rate for a given number living at each age-period. In figure 2 a comparison is given of the experience of

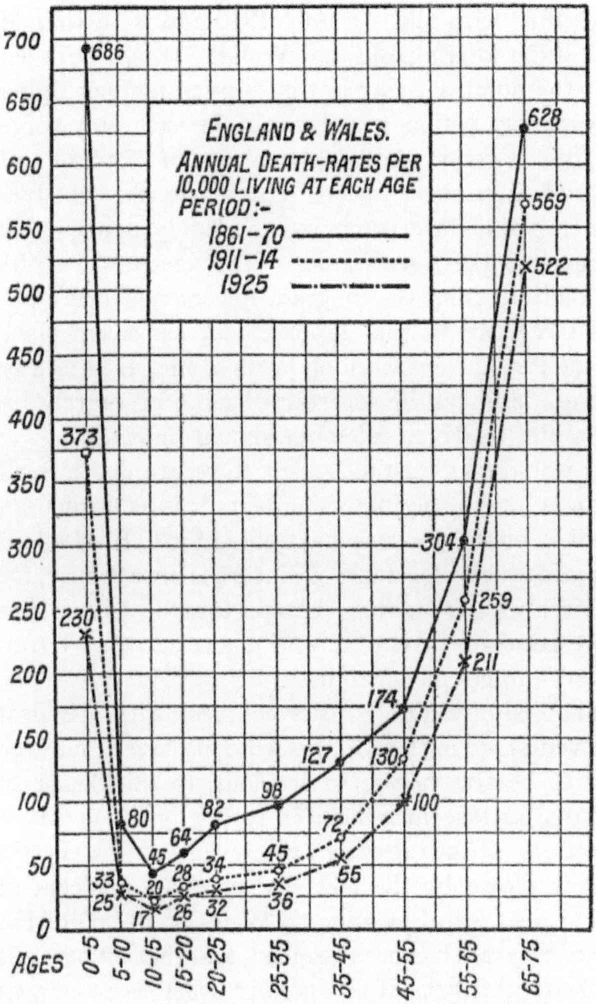
ENGLAND & WALES.
ANNUAL DEATH-RATES PER 10,000 LIVING AT EACH AGE PERIOD:-
1861-70
1911-14
1925
700
650
600
550
500
450
400
350
300
250
200
150
100
50
0
686
628
569
522
373
304
259
230
211
174
127
130
98
100
82
80
64
72
45
45
34
28
33
20
55
25
17
26
32
36
AGES
0-5
5-10
10-15
15-20
20-25
25-35
35-45
45-55
55-65
65-75

FIG. 2

1861–1870 with that of 1907–1910 and with that of 1911–1920 for England and Wales. It will be seen that the number dying out of a given number living at each age-period has declined in each successive decade. Even at the advanced ages of 75 to 85 and 85 to 95 there was a lowered death rate when the two earlier periods are compared, and only a negligible increase in the last decade. (The ages of 75 to 85 are omitted from the diagram for convenience.)

A large part of this improvement has taken place during the efficient working years of life, as is seen in figure 2, and can be ascertained more accurately by life-tables to which reference should be made.

It would be a mistaken view to regard death itself as an evil. In the fulness of years it is as normal an event as birth. As Goethe (quoted by T. H. Huxley) has said: "The spectacle of Nature is always new, for she is always renewing the spectators. Life is her most exquisite invention, and death her expert contrivance to get plenty of life."

The real objection is to premature death, which if the widest definition of the word be given, may be said to be always due to accident, to suicide, or to external maleficent influences especially the germs of infection. That the extent of preventive work is still vast is shown by the fact that some 64 per cent of all the deaths in England and Wales occur before the age of 65 years has been reached, and that 39 per cent of the total deaths at all ages occur between the ages of 15 and 65, the working years of life. As we proceed it will be seen how vast is the number of these which are preventible. Although our knowledge of prevention in many respects is still defective, our knowledge is immensely greater than our practical application of this knowledge.

# CHAPTER II

## Causation of Disease

Although it would appear more orderly to describe first the growth of our knowledge as to the physiological and physical aspects of personal health, this discussion is postponed to later chapters, as our best knowledge of these aspects of health is of recent date.

In Chapter VIII of *Evolution of Preventive Medicine* some account is given of the beginning of our knowledge of the causation of some of the chief epidemic plagues of mankind. In Chapter IX of the same volume were outlined earlier views of the causes of pandemicity and of the "epidemic constitution," while in Chapter XI outstanding points in the history of contagium vivum were given. The relation of this doctrine to typhus was stated in Chapter XIII; and in Chapters XV and XVI the stages of disentanglement of "fever" into typhus and enteric fevers were outlined.

Snow was the father of the doctrine of specificity of infection in England, as Bretonneau was in France. Snow's marvellous insight into the true causation of cholera and typhoid fever has been brought out in Chapter XVII of *Evolution of Preventive Medicine*. The beginnings of the possibility of prevention of non-specific infection in parturition have been described in Chapter XX of the same volume. Thus far have some of the stages in the elucidation of infectious diseases been stated; but it appears desirable to add here further remarks on the evolution of our knowledge of these diseases.

Successive plausible explanations of their occurrence have held the minds of men, and the progress of medicine and especially of preventive medicine has only been made possible by the demolition of these erroneous though plausible views by carefully ascertained experience, and in more recent years also by experimentation.

Hippocrates in his *De Morbis* advised that none should presume to treat diseases that have not first well considered their causes: wise counsel, but then almost impossible to follow, for treatment was urgently called for, and investigation of causation was slow and dubious in result. Hence hypothesis and doctrine naturally replaced science as the guide to treatment.

Two methods of advance in knowledge of the nature of disease emerged, the experiential and the experimental. The first is naturally associated with the name of Sydenham who wrote:

> I have often thought that if we had an exact history of every disease, we should never want a remedy suitable to it.

Lord Verulam (Francis Bacon) had much to say also on this method of investigating disease. Thus:

> The capital things of nature generally lie out of the beaten paths: . . . . And here let none despair, or be confounded,

if the experiments they attempt should not answer their expectation: for though success be indeed more pleasing; yet failure, frequently is no less informing . . . . He therefore and only he deserveth the name of a good physician who always deduces his curative indications from the cause of the disease . . . . (*De Augment Scient.*, sec. xii).

Of one cause of disease Bacon himself had no doubt, concluding with close approximation to truth that

Gluttony . . . in regard to its frequency and pernicious effects ought to be placed foremost of all the antecedents of acute diseases.

One might continue indefinitely culling from medical pronouncements as to disease causation, and one more may be added in illustration of the gropings and stumblings of the past. Thackrah on page 66 of his well-known work wrote:

If a man suffer today from headache and sickness, the effect of yesterday's debauch, he ascribes them to the cold he took in returning home. If his bowels be irritable from the annoyance of undigested aliment, he has "taken cold." If he suffer from an epidemic, he is sure it arose from "sitting with his back to an open window." . . . . Nay, the unhappy victim of hereditary consumption, ascribes his illness to "sleeping in a damp bed."

There is sound sense in the greater part of Thackrah's statement, though the reference to phthisis illustrates how the doctrine of one century may, with the growth of knowledge, be relegated to the "scrap heap" in the next.

The stage of evolution in which study of the natural history of disease was the chief means of determining its nature and causation (see *Nosography* by Kund Faber, 1923) was followed by the sedulous study of diseased organs in autopsies of which Morgagni's work in 1760 is outstanding. Morgagni regarded such study as conducing to a knowledge of the causation of disease, for the full title of his treatise was "De sedibus *et causis* Morborum per signa diagnostica investigatis et per anatomen confirmatis." Various nosologies of disease appeared, and Linnœus described symptoms as having the same relation to a disease as leaves to the plant from which they spring. Laennec, who died aged 45 in 1821, initiated the examination as well as the observation of each patient (by the stethoscope) thus laying the foundation of ante-mortem pathology, as Morgagni had done for post-mortem pathology. He first divined the fact that all stages of tuberculosis constitute a single disease; he also accurately described emphysema, acute œdema of the lung, bronchiectasis and lung gangrene.

The conception of unification in tuberculosis was one of the earliest approaches to knowledge of specificity of disease; and around the conception of specificity has centered the struggle between different views of causation which in some measure still continues.

Bretonneau's name stands out with that of Laennec as a protagonist of specificity. He first described diphtheritic angina and croup as an etiological and clinical entity; and as Faber remarks "since Bretonneau the specificity of diseases has in fact always been implied." He controverted the argument based on the membranous character of the inflammation produced by the application of extract of cantharides, by showing that, although this membrane resembles that of diphtheria, the clinical course pursued in the two cases differs entirely.

Bretonneau also advocated the view that the intestinal lesions in enteric fever are specific in character (see *Traités de la Dothientérie et de la Spécificité*, published from Bretonneau's original Manuscripts, 1922), and he propounded the hypothesis that both diphtheria and dothientérie develope "under the influence of a contagious principle . . . . a reproductive element" which was comparable to an intestinal parasite. But he carefully safeguarded himself against the erroneous conception still too common that contagia constitute the diseases: "les maladies ne sont pas des êtres."

The doctrine of specificity was controverted by Broussais, who described his own doctrine as "physiological medicine," and attached more importance to functional disorders of diseased organs than to their anatomical changes. Of course neither view was adequate.

Traversing Laennec's teaching as to the specificity of tuberculosis, Broussais regarded this as like the older ontological view that diseases, like plants, are special beings. In objecting to this view he was right; and the reminder that all disease entities are abstract concepts created in man's mind remains relevant. It is, as Faber has pointed out, equally true for botanical and zoological species, in which nevertheless enumeration and classification are indispensable. The concept is necessary, but its limitations must be realized.

The separation of disease from disease continued steadily as an indispensable part of progress; and so by combination of clinical and anatomical investigation, various diseases were differentiated. Thus Bright elucidated the nature of chronic renal disease, Addison of suprarenal disease; and in more recent years many pathological entities have been discovered, and, with their isolation from other diseases presenting somewhat similar symptoms, the way has been pointed to etiological inquiry and thus to preventive measures.

The German school of medicine in which Virchow's fame stands foremost, attempted to ascertain by physiological experiment and otherwise the interrelation and development of the phenomena of disease. This school in Faber's words "from the beginning resisted every endeavour to establish definite clinical pictures, or to describe individual diseases." Every mention of specific character was "opposed and dubbed ontology." Virchow is also quoted by Faber as saying in 1848, "Nowadays ontology is again attempting to creep into therapy in all sorts of disguises as we see it most markedly in the so-called specific methods of cure."

Virchow's further statement that "disease is nothing but life under altered conditions" is acceptable; but his plea against ontological therapy is less so, in view of modern therapeutics and particularly in the light of the increasing triumphs of chemo-therapeutics, as for instance arseno-benzol preparations for syphilis, and allied compounds in the treatment of rat-bite fever, of relapsing fever, yaws, sleeping sickness, etc.

Virchow's cellular pathology has done less for the progress of curative and preventive medicine than accurate study of clinical medicine and pathology. Microscopic examination suggested that the miliary tubercle and the caseous products in tuberculosis are of different origin: and it was because of this erroneous pathological view that Niemeyer made this famous pronouncement: "The greatest evil which can happen to a consumptive is that he should become tuberculous."

Even Villemin's demonstration in 1865 that tubercle could be inoculated into animals by caseous as well as by miliary tubercle did not shake this doctrine. A similar dualism was taught for diphtheria and croup; and indeed all doctrinal teaching of specificity was denounced.

On the other hand Trousseau represented both English and French medicine when he said: "To know the natural cause of the diseases is more than one-half of medicine." He was equally emphatic on the specific character of disease:

> This important question dominates all pathology, all medicine, in a word, all medical science. The natural history of the diseases resembles that of the animals and plants; it deals, in the same way, with specific properties which separate the species.

The physiological school in its opposition to specificity was, however, preparing the way to a more comprehensive knowledge of medicine. The discovery of methods of counting blood cells, of the sphymograph and ophthalmoscope (1850) of the laryngoscope (1854 and 1857) and such investigations as those of Claude Bernard on glycosuria were opening the way to a vast extension of experimental medicine to pathology.

Many discoveries must be credited to the school of thought which denied the specificity of specific diseases, and which regarded it as an adequate explanation of disease to state that it is function in abnormal conditions. The discovery in 1869 of chloral hydrate by Liebreich was followed by the finding of other hypnotics and of various anti-febrile and anti-neuralgic drugs. Then followed the discovery of local anaesthetics, cocaine in 1884, and later stovain and others.

The specific treatment of specific diseases had greater triumphs to show as will be seen later.

In Pasteur's fundamental experiments there came

the revelation of the true nature of the specificity which Sydenham, Bretonneau, Laennec, Trousseau and many others had championed, and the perpetual craving for so called "ontology" was in large measure justified. The new knowledge made it possible to consider every disease from an *etiological standpoint.* Koch may be said to have abolished Virchow; and in this connection the following statement by Wunderlich writing in 1859 is interesting:

> Sydenham's vagueness of thought deluded him into ideas which led his successors to take the wrong paths. To such ideas belong his postulates concerning a distinct nomenclature and specification of the different forms of diseases, and his delusion that specific remedies may be found for all or most diseases. (Quoted by K. Faber in "Nosography," p. 109.)

The final proof of the doctrine of specificity in its application to infectious diseases is furnished by the specific curative and preventive treatment discovered by following its teaching.

Quinine in malaria is the first example of this, ascertained empirically. So also the value of mercury in syphilis was thus ascertained. The more recent triumphs of chemotherapy can only be mentioned. Ehrlich's salvarsan (606) in vitro does not kill the spirochetes responsible for syphilis, but it attacks the parasite selectively in the living tissues of the infected person; and for other diseases due to trypanosomes it has been shown to be practicable to intervene by appropriate eliotropic remedies (so called by Meyer and Gottlieb) to intervene in the struggle between the invading microbes and the body cells, and either destroy the former or place them *hors de combat.*

The position now attained, which year by year is being consolidated and extended, is well summarized in a statement by Fr. Müller (1905) quoted by Faber (loc. cit, p. 162):

> The attempt to class and name the diseases according to their etiology and not according to their pathologico-anatomical base has not only proved beneficial in the field of infectious diseases but has *inter alia* given excellent results in the case of heart diseases. It will also be permissible to apply the principle of division to the nephritic diseases.

Our recent additions to the therapeutics of diseases of the ductless glands forms another important chapter in the history of specificity. (See Chapter XXIV for thyroid disease.)

But the most important outcome of knowledge of the specific causation of infectious diseases,—confirming the earlier empirical success of vaccination against small pox,—is seen in the treatment of rabies by Pasteur's method, in the prevention of typhoid fever by anti-typhoid serum, in the similar case of cholera, in the immunity against diphtheria secured by administration of its toxoid-antitoxin, and in other similar cases to which reference is made in later pages.

We are now in a more favorable position for considering what causes disease. It is evident that a given function may become abnormal as the result of more than one factor, acting together or separately; and it is evident also that one cannot properly speak of disorder, even when it has resulted in organic changes in normal tissues, as an actual entity, distinguishable from the patient himself. But one can fairly regard all the consequences of the operation of poisons developed as the result of physiological disorder or due to a given invading agent, whether it be a chemical poison like phosphorus or lead, or a microbe like the anthrax bacillus, as an entity without offending against reason or entertaining a conception which is unsound.

Very often a single agent cannot be regarded as a cause, and we more appropriately speak of a series of conditions conducing to disease. A spark will fire a train of gunpowder, and an avalanche may be precipitated by a shout; but in each instance many prior factors are involved. In the instances named we should all give a more important place to the spark than to the human voice; but in relation to the causation of certain infectious diseases, especially of tuberculosis, the relative importance of soil (*le terrain*) and of seed (*le microbe*) is likely to continue for long to be the subject of research and of difference of opinion. In tuberculosis the persistent tendency to minimise the importance of "seed" and to exaggerate the need for concentrating a "soil," appears to me to darken counsel.

# CHAPTER III

## The Earlier Work of Pasteur and His Predecessors

To know the circumstances in which a given infectious disease prevails excessively is most helpful in its prevention. Hence the great value of studies of disease in relation to inimical industrial and social circumstances, and of its more general epidemiology. But these methods of study could not in most instances functify in successful preventive measures until the doctrine of contagium vivum had been established on a firm basis. Prior to Pasteur this doctrine, even when held, was usually associated with the notion that the disease in question might also arise autocthonously, i.e., *de novo*. Without denying the evolution of pathogenicity in innocent microbes under unknown conditions, it is now accepted that the success of preventive measures against our chief infectious diseases depends on the assumption of specific pathogenicity of a special microbe for each disease. The notion that any specific infection can, at least occasionally, arise *de novo* held good so long as spontaneous generation of contagia or other lowly organized living cells was regarded as possible.

Louis Pasteur was born in 1822 and died in 1895. The story of his life and work can be read in S.

Paget's elementary sketch *Pasteur and After Pasteur*, 1914, in M. Vallery Radot's *Vie de Pasteur*, translated into English by Wm. Devonshire, and in Descour's *Pasteur and His Work* translated into English by Dr. B. H. Webb, 1922. Pasteur's earlier investigations on crystallography were followed in 1856 by a study of the problems of fermentation. Prior to his time this had been regarded as a purely chemical process, the general view formulated by Liebig being that "beer yeast, and in general all the animal and vegetable substances in a state of putrefaction, convey to other bodies the state of decomposition in which they are themselves."

True, Leeuenhoeck in 1689 had discovered under the microscope ovoid globules apparently organised, and in 1835 Cagniard de la Tour had made the same observation. The last named showed that yeast was a mass of globules capable of reproduction by budding, and he regarded it as probable that as a result of the growth of these globules, carbonic acid was set free from sugar and alcohol produced. But the view commonly taken and voiced by Berzelius was that these globules "were merely a chemical product, a precipitate formed during the fermentation;" while Liebig regarded the absence of these globules in analogous fermentations, e.g., the lactic, as a proof of the insignificance of their rôle.

This being the state of scientific opinion, Pasteur intermitted his studies of alcoholic fermentation in order to ascertain whether a yeast was or was not concerned in lactic fermentation; and it was in this investigation that he first employed the process of "sowing" and repeatedly sowing a minute trace of the veil of yeast of this fermenting liquid into a new solution and thus setting up fresh fermentation, which made subsequent progress in bacteriology possible. The great step forward made by him was enunciated in the words: "fermentation is thus shown to be correlated to the life and formation of the globules, and not to their death or putrefaction": and that it furthermore was not a result of mere contact, but that interchange of substance occurred.

These and allied investigations obviously raised the problem as to the origin of ferments; and this meant a reconsideration of the perennial problem of spontaneous generation (heterogenesis).

St. Paul's statement "Thou fool, that which thou sowest is not quickened except it die," embodies a profound truth in the generation of seeds, but the extremes to which the belief in spontaneous generation went among the ancients and mediaevalists is shown by Van Helmont's recipe for procuring rats (quoted in Descour's *Pasteur and His Work*):

> Cork up a pot containing corn with a dirty shirt; after about 21 days a ferment coming from the dirty shirt combines with the effluvium from the wheat, the grains of which are turned into rats.

To Francesco Redi, an Italian naturalist who died about 1650, is due the credit of repudiating spontaneous generation, and disproving it in a particular instance. He exposed fresh meat under fine gauze and thus kept it free from maggots; and he may be regarded as the father of the doctrine of *biogenesis*. He had, as Huxley remarked in a lecture in 1870, to pay the customary tax on a discoverer, of defending himself against the charge of impugning the veracity of the Scriptures; for is it not written that "out of the eater came forth meat, and out of the strong came forth sweetness?"

It is true that Harvey, a contemporary of Redi, had enunciated the aphorism *omne vivum ex ovo;* he believed that every living thing comes from an egg, but added "or from the dissolved elements of anterior life." The view embodied in the last quoted words appeared to be confirmed by Needham's experiments in the eighteenth century. He showed that decomposition took place in the contents of vessels, which had been subjected to the temperature of cooking; and Needham's views were accepted by Buffon, who held that " . . . . the matter of living beings preserves after death some of its vitality."

In 1765 Spallanzani criticised Needham's results, which did not coincide with his own. He affirmed that Needham's corks were inefficient, and that he had not subjected his flagons to a sufficiently high temperature.

Pasteur in February, 1860, reported his first results on spontaneous generation to the Academy of Science. The classical experiments in which he succeeded in keeping saccharine and other fluids in flasks free from decomposition are well known. He used sterilized cotton wool plugs, and he succeeded also without plugs by having a glass tube communicating with the interior of the flask and with the external air, but with a deep U-shaped bend in it. The details of his experiments may be read in the above works (page 24) and in his great "Memoire sur les corpuscles organisés qui existent dans l'atmosphere" (*Ann. de Chimie et de Physique*, 1862, lxiv). Strained air did not develop life in fluids; germs could be found among the solid parts of the strainer; that these were capable of producing fermentation was shown by sowing them in a solution fitted for their development; and similar deposits, could be discovered in the bent tubes which had prevented a decomposable liquid from decomposing.

Pasteur's demonstration was not, however, regarded by all as conclusive; and in England Tyndall for and Bastian against Pasteur's conclusion carried on the controversy for some years. Tyndall showed by beautiful experiments that "ordinary air is not better than a sort of stirabout of excessively minute solid particles," and that air can be rendered optically pure by heat or by straining through cotton wool.

There was some difficulty in accepting Pasteur's general conclusions enunciated at the Sorbonne in April, 1864: "Under no condition known today can we affirm that microscopic beings come into the world without germs, without parents of their own nature."

This difficulty arose from Bastian's experiment showing that in urine which had been boiled and made alkaline, fermentation occurred when the sealed flask was kept in an incubator at 122°F. (50°C.). Further investigations by Pasteur showed, however, that certain bacteria, especially the *Bacillus subtilis*, form spores which resist the temperature of boiling (212°F. or 100°C.); but that the growth of any such organisms in a solution which had been subjected for half an hour to a temperature of 120°C. could be prevented, if the flask in which this experiment was made had while dry been previously exposed to dry heat at 120°C. The fact that dry air is completely sterilized at this temperature has made possible modern refinements of antiseptic surgery; and this, like the analogous facts bearing on the doctrine of specificity (page 20), has given final confirmation to the absence of spontaneous generation under any known present conditions. In this connection may be quoted two dicta of Pasteur the truth of which science has repeatedly confirmed. "The characteristic of erroneous theories is the impossibility of foreseeing new facts. . . . . The characteristic of a true theory is its fruitfulness."

# CHAPTER IV

## The First and Greatest Triumph in Application of the Germ Theory

Through the ages wounds have been dangerous to an extent which it is now difficult to realize. Erysipelas or some other septic infection has been the continual dread of surgeons. They have approached, on their account, even minor operations with trepidation.

Sir James Paget in addressing the British Medical Association in 1862 urged the study of pyœmic diseases. He spoke of the "deep regrets, the bitter disappointments from which we might be saved if there were less risks" in operations; and referred also to the "tolerated barbarisms of practice," only justified by the belief that the risk of "a cutting operation is so great that there is nothing too bad to be substituted for it." So late as 1876 a skilful surgeon, seeing the terrible mortality after operations in hospitals, declared that he never wished to touch a knife again. Another surgeon advised looking at the operating knife ten times before taking it up, for if an operation were decided on, it often meant signing a death-warrant.

The air in hospitals was regarded as almost necessarily maleficent, the unsuccessful surgeon blaming the architect: and it is not surprising that Sir Jas. Simpson and Florence Nightingale alike regarded hospitals as enemies to life and health.

John Bell writing of hospital gangrene early in the nineteenth century said "this is a hospital disease; without the circle of the infected walls the men are safe;" and in 1812 he stated that abdominal wounds were so generally fatal that it was only necessary to record the result in the extraordinary cases that recovered! Compound fractures were fatal in from a quarter to three-fifths of the total cases; and limbs were ruthlessly sacrificed as involving much smaller risk than conservative surgery. But in the Franco-German War 1870–1871 some 13,000 amputations were recorded by the French of which 10,000 were fatal.

In 1864 Sir Spencer Wells in an address to the British Medical Association quoted with favour the statement made in the French Academy of Medicine that the mortality from erysipelas and allied affections associated with overcrowding increased when surgical wards were over medical wards. In the same address Wells quoted Pasteur's recent experiments on the filtration of germs from air, and drew deductions as to the importance of pure air in hospital wards; but it was left for Lister to search diligently for methods of protecting each individual wound from aerial contamination. Modern surgery, it may be added, owes much to Wells' pioneer work on ovariotomy; attempts were made to prevent the operation at certain hospitals, as endangering the character of the profession.

Joseph Lister was born in 1827 and died in 1902. In 1861 he was appointed on the surgical staff of the Glasgow Infirmary, and there his work, which revolutionized surgery, began. At that time the surgical wards of the Infirmary were ravaged by surgical pyœmia and hospital gangrene. The introduction of anaesthetics, beneficent in itself, had served to increase the hospital mortality by rendering a larger number of operations possible. But although this for the time being was true, it is none the less noteworthy that between 1811 and 1827 were born Pasteur, Lister, and Simpson, who with the discoverers of ether have made the triumphs of modern surgery possible.

Anaesthesia as a necessary link in the greatest triumph of preventive and curative medicine deserves more than a passing reference. Humphrey Davy, born in 1778, described nitrous oxide, and when only aged 21 wrote of its anaesthetic properties. A demonstration of these properties was made in Guy's Hospital, London; but its wonderful potentialities appear to have been unperceived. It was not until 1844 that the first tooth was extracted under "gas" by Dr. Horace Wells at Hartford, Connecticut. In October 1846 ether was first successfully administered in Boston Massachusetts by Warren and Morton; and in 1847 Simpson published his paper, on "Account of a new anaesthetic agent, as a substitute for sulphuric ether in surgery and midwifery." This paper bore the appropriate inscription from Bacon "I esteem it the office of the Physician not only to restore health, but to mitigate pain and dolours." At the dates named above it was very imperfectly realised how vastly anaesthesia was to increase the possibilities of cure of disease and prevention of its complications.

When appointed at Glasgow, Lister had already devoted much study to the causes of inflammation and suppuration; and he had come to the tentative conclusion that pus is formed in wounds as the result of irritation of the granulation tissue which covers the raw surface. He also regarded the putrefaction of the discharges in the wound as the most probable irritative agent, and considered that putrefaction is due to something which comes from without. The absence of suppuration in serious injuries in which the skin remained unbroken appeared to him most significant.

He satisfied himself that exclusion of air was not responsible for freedom from suppuration. Thus in fracture of the ribs, in which the lung was punctured, air from within the lungs did not set up an empyema. Hence something sometimes was conveyed by air, which at other times was excluded, and this something set up decomposition.

Lister's first efforts were directed not to the exclusion of this "something," but especially to methods which would secure cleanliness of surgical technique and of wounds, and thus inhibit decomposition. Antiseptics had already been used in washing wounds, and Lister experimented with them, and especially with Condy's fluid. No great success was achieved.

But after having had his attention drawn to Pasteur's paper already quoted (page 27) in which, as Lister himself said in an address delivered 32 years later, it was shown that "putrefaction was a fermentation caused by the growth of microbes, and that these could not arise *de novo* in the decomposable substances," the problem assumed a more hopeful aspect.

This was in 1864. Lister found that Pasteur's recent papers contained the clue to the practical prevention of sepsis. The enemy was not a gas present everywhere, but solid particles "capable of being killed or avoided" (Cheyne). At once Lister darted straight to the fundamental conclusion in preventive medicine as applied to surgery, that external germs must be prevented from getting into wounds and if possible must be destroyed outside the wound.

The various methods by means of which matter producing putrefaction was prevented more or less successfully from entering and multiplying in a wound need not be described here.

The author remembers the years 1878–1880 when in St. Thomas's Hospital, London, the carbolic spray constantly directed over a wound during an operation was regarded as an essential part of the needed precautions. Gradually as experience increased, it became clear that the germs floating in the air had relatively small significance, and that minute particles of "dirt" in the surgeon's or nurses' finger nails or hands, or on the various instruments employed in the operation, and the lack of complete asepsis in ligatures, especially ligatures for arteries, or in dressings for the wound, were chief sources of danger. So rapidly did this view extend that an attempt was made to describe a separate school of asepticism, as distinguished from antisepticism; and some surgeons showed remarkably good operative results, especially in abdominal operations where reliance was placed on boiled water, boiled instruments, and scrupulously clean hands and dressings as safeguards against sepsis. The distinction is almost fatuous, for the essential principle of Listerism is merely that some effective method shall be adopted for securing the freedom of wounds from pathogenic germs introduced from without.

T. H. Huxley in an address to the British Association 1870 summed up the position with accuracy; though no one at that date could realize the phenomenal saving of life which the universal adoption of Lister's surgical principles would secure:

It seems to me impossible to rise from the perusal of Professor Lister's publication on the antiseptic method of treatment without a strong conviction that the lamentable mortality which so frequently dogs the footsteps of the most skilled operator, and those deadly consequences of wounds and injuries which seem to haunt the very walls of great hospitals, and are, even now, destroying more men than die of bullet or bayonet, are due to the importation of minute organisms into wounds, and their increase and multiplication; and that the surgeon who saves most lives will be he who best works out the practical consequences of the hypothesis of Redi.

Koch, possibly stimulated by the surgical calamities of the Franco-German war, in which the mortality from gunshot wounds was terrible, concluded in 1878 a bacteriological examination of the pathology of wounds which justified Listerism, and placed its method on a basis of experimentally ascertained facts.

The general principle underlying Lister's method of dressing wounds is that by its means an open wound is practically converted into a subcutaneous wound, so far as external infection is concerned. This can sometimes be secured by exact bacteriological cleanliness in operations; but,—and especially in complicated septic wounds in warfare,—this is often impossible, and antisepsis by chemical agents is also required.

At the present time Listerism has triumphed in every branch of surgery. It has not, however, come to fruition in midwifery. In this branch of medicine, as seen in Chapter XX of my *Evolution of Preventive Medicine*, Semmelweiss had in some measure anticipated Lister's methods; but in private obstetric practice they still commonly fail to be adopted.

Owing to the relative safety of drastic operations rendered possible by Listerism, the scope of cure of disease has been vastly extended. Earlier operations are now performed, the number of inoperable diseases has been gradually decreased, and surgery has also proved itself an important instrument of research, as for instance in the elucidation of the functions of parts of the nervous system.

# CHAPTER V

## Earlier Discoveries in Bacteriology

When Pasteur's earlier work led to the discovery that fermentation meant the multiplication of minute organisms in an appropriate fluid, he could not have anticipated that in 1897 Buchner would extract from yeast its ferment, zymose, formed within the yeast cells just as ptyalin is formed within the cells of the salivary glands; and that thus there would be effected a reconcilement between Liebig who thought of fermentation as a problem in molecular physics and Pasteur who regarded it in terms of plant physiology (page 27). Pasteur's remarkable work showing that in all known conditions life alone originates life (La vie c'est le germe et le germe c'est la vie"), naturally led him to the flight of speculative vision which was always inciting him to further experimentation. In 1863 he informed the French Emperor that his one ambition was to ascertain the causes of putrid and contagious diseases; and as early as 1860 writing of his experiments on the sterility of the air at Chamonix above the snow level, he regarded his observations as "preparing the way for a thorough study of the origin of different diseases."

I do not propose to follow Pasteur's research on pébrine, a decimating disease of silkworms, which formed his first introduction to pathological research.

These researches began in 1865 and lasted some six years. Towards the end of 1867 he had solved the problem and was in a position to give exact instructions to silk worm breeders. The story of the means by which Pasteur traced the process of infection in the successive stages of development of the moth and discovered how to separate the infected from the non-infected worms need not be detailed here. Complications occurred owing to the occurrence of a second disease, flachery, and in investigating this and pébrine Pasteur came across facts which opened up in his mind the notion of an increase of virulence in passing from one organism to another. It also appeared that virulence might vary according to the route of entry of the virus, and that devitalising factors might reduce resistance to infection. Here were the intellectual germs of some of Pasteur's later researches.

At this time there were two schools of thought as to bacteria and disease. Darwin's *Origin of Species* had been published and the principle of evolution seemed to point to pleomorphism, i.e., rapid change of species in these lowly microörganisms. In the light of his own investigations Pasteur was convinced that each germ was specific, and that each fermentation had its own specific ferment. Lister ranged himself at first with the pleomorphists; though when the discoveries rendered possible by Koch's improved technique had been made, he adopted the opposite view. His words deserve quotation: "Next to the promulgation of truth, the best thing I can conceive that a man can do is the recantation of a published error." He himself, before Koch's methods became available, succeeded in growing a pure cultivation of "*Bacterium lactis*" in sterile milk, using a modification of Pasteur's method of minute division of preceding growths. Gradually Pasteur's views and those which in 1872 F. Cohn systematised prevailed; and they were the real starting points for the study of methods for cultivation of bacteria in a pure state.

As early as 1857 Pasteur had grown bacteria in liquids, and then by multiple sowings had increased the purity of his cultures. But these were always open to slight suspicion; and Koch doubted the purity of Pasteur's later cultures of anthrax bacilli. The marvel is that, depending as he did solely on multiple dilutions in liquid media, Pasteur was able to obtain his great results.

To remedy these difficulties of technique various attempts were made; and the problem was solved by Robert Koch (1843–1910), who rightly stands side by side with Pasteur as a founder of modern bacteriology. Beginning first with hanging drop methods, and then employing growths of bacteria on sliced potatoes, he gradually (in 1883) evolved the method of adding the inoculated material to melted gelatine and then pouring it on a cooled glass plate. He thus secured isolated pure growths on the solid gelatine, which could easily be sub-cultured. In 1878 the use of agar agar was introduced. There followed a rapid succession of discoveries of the causal organisms of infectious diseases; and, as Bulloch has put it, the decade 1878–1886 was the heyday of bacteriological etiological discovery, while the decade 1886–1896 became the first great period of immunological research.

1880 Koch worked out the causes of several traumatic diseases in animals
1882 Koch discovered the tubercle bacillus
1884 Koch discovered the cholera vibrio
1882 Lœffler and Schütz isolated the glanders bacillus
1882 Gaffky isolated the typhoid bacillus
1884 Lœffler isolated the diphtheria bacillus

Later reference will be made to some of the above discoveries; here, before giving an outline of the work of Pasteur and Koch on anthrax, it appears desirable to revert to the subject of the two schools of bacteriological thought mentioned on page 38.

In the light of recent investigations and speculations, and in view of apparent teaching of epidemiology, are we to revert to the older view, which in its crudest stage held for instance, that the hay bacillus (*B. subtilis*) can become the anthrax bacillus, that a common field bacillus may be the progenitor of the tubercle bacillus, or that the common colon bacillus developes into the typhoid bacillus of Eberth? There is no inherent improbability in such a view. The life-history of the microbe as well as of the host is concerned; and variations in either may produce differences in the reaction between the two. But although this is so, we need to restrain exuberance of imagination in this connection. Whatever, may happen in the slow course of the ages, the steady specificity of some of the chief infective microörganisms is well established. No one now expects a case of typhus to be autochthonously originated; and a similar scepticism is entertained for typhoid fever. Origin *de novo* would be stoutly denied by all for rabies, or anthrax or syphilis. On the other hand changes in both virulence and infectivity are seen in the epidemiological history of smallpox, scarlet fever and of influenza and its congeners, however we may incline to explain them.

### ANTHRAX

Anthrax both in animals and in man is a deadly disease. In man it occurs in two chief forms, malignant pustule, from inoculation of infective matter derived from the hides or blood of animals suffering from anthax; and pneumonia, commonly known as "wool sorter's disease," because in the absence of adequate precautions it occurs in those handling alpaca and other foreign sheep's hides or the wool from them. Malignant pustule has been caused by shaving with a shaving brush, the bristles of which were derived from an animal suffering from anthrax.

The story of the work of Pasteur and Koch on anthrax is that of a potential triumph over infection which is only less striking than the triumph over wound infections secured by Lister's work.

Pollender in 1849 had observed minute rod-shaped bodies in the blood of animals suffering from anthrax. Davaine in 1861 accurately described the *Bacillus anthracis*, and later he showed that the virulence of the disease showed some proportion to the number of bacteria present. By inoculation experiments Klebs in 1879 showed that the serum of filtered blood did not produce anthrax. Davaine had previously shown that the *Bacillus anthracis* disappeared from the tissues of an infected animal during putrefaction, but that blood which had been dried quickly retained its virulence a long time.

In tracing the events which enabled the life history of the anthrax and other bacilli to be satisfactorily investigated, a preliminary necessary step was the discovery of Weigert in 1871 that bacteria can be differentiated by special stains. He began in 1875 to use anilin dyes for this purpose.

From 1871 onwards, Robert Koch, who in that year was 28 years old and engaged in general medical practice in East Prussia, began as an amateur to make microscopic examination of various tissues. With rapidly increasing skill he felt his way, and happening to examine the blood of sheep which had died of anthrax, he concentrated on the examination of the minute rods visible in the blood of these animals.

Like Davaine he found that they were consistently absent from the blood of healthy animals, and always present in the blood of animals presenting the symptoms of this terrible disease. As sheep were too dear for his work, he inoculated mice with the specifically contaminated blood. For this purpose he employed small pieces of wood previously heated in an oven and then smeared with the infected sheep's blood, the wood being inserted into a clean cut at the root of the mouse's tail. Mice thus treated soon died and presented the characteristic spleen and black blood of infected sheep. The same bacilli were present in this blood, and when watched under the microscope they increased in size and multiplied manifold. Hence they were alive.

Koch then considered how he might watch the growth of these microörganisms. After various efforts, he employed the aqueous humor of an ox's eye kept approximately at the body temperature, and devised the "hanging drop" method, the drop being inverted on a cover glass over a concave well in a larger slide and protected from contamination. This was carried on through seven or eight generations; and some of the final liquid inoculated into a mouse's tail, again reproduced the disease showing the same symptoms and the characteristic bacilli.

This was the first demonstration of the causal relation of a pathogenic bacillus to a specific disease; and it fulfilled all the conditions of what are known as Koch's postulates. These may be thus summarised:

1. The assumed pathogenic organism is found in each case in the morbid lesions of the disease.

2. It is not found in any other disease, except out of relation to any morbid conditions.
3. It can be isolated from the diseased body.
4. It can be sub-cultured.
5. It can be inoculated into another animal producing the same disease.
6. The same organism can be recovered from this animal.

Pasteur had blazed the path in bacteriology; Koch made it a highway, along which it became practicable to travel towards the ideal time already prophesied by Pasteur when it would be "within the power of man to make parasitic diseases disappear from the face of the earth." In 1877 Pasteur using liquid media showed that cultures could be carried on by minute sowings of anthrax bacilli to the hundredth generation, maintaining the specific character of this organism.

To complete the story, the steps by which spores were demonstrated must be stated. How was it that in certain pastures (*champs maudits*) no flock could be kept without some animals falling victims to anthrax?

Pasteur in 1860 had showed that a temperature higher than 100°C. is required to kill some organisms, and in 1869 he demonstrated the presence of resistant bodies in flachery.

Koch ascertained that when a smear of anthrax blood was allowed to dry on glass and kept thus for a couple of days, no disease resulted if water was added and the mixture was inoculated into small animals.

He then watched a hanging drop containing anthrax bacilli which was kept for a day at the temperature of a mouse's body. The bacilli when now examined showed threads which were speckled with ovals, like a string of pearls. That these beads were spores was verified by further experiments including the taking of a spleen from an infected animal which was then incubated at 100°C. These and later experiments showed that spores were not formed in the living host, and that access to oxygen was necessary for their formation.

# CHAPTER VI

## Earlier Attempts at Specific Prophylaxis

The medical mind has always been occupied with the problem as to why a person who has recovered from an attack of measles, or scarlet fever, or yellow fever, or of many other infectious diseases seldom suffers from a second attack, when exposed to infection. This problem exercised Pasteur's mind, and his thoughts necessarily were influenced by the classical instance furnished by the protective influence of vaccinia against smallpox (see *Evolution of Preventive Medicine*, Chapter XIX). This instance at once suggests at least two methods of immunisation.

(1) By a prior attack of the disease in question, or
(2) As in the case of small pox by the inoculation of the virus of a closely allied disease, which however, differs in that its manifestation is limited to the place of inoculation.

The result in either case was regarded as explicable on the older view, held by Pasteur and others, that some material in the body tissues necessary for producing the disease has been permanently removed or reduced; and in support of this view the case of alcoholic fermentation can be cited. This ceases in a saccharine solution when 12 or 13 per cent of alcohol has accumulated, even though the sugar is not exhausted.

In 1879 Pasteur had already succeeded in growing more or less uncontaminated cultures of specific organisms in fluid media. His next supremely important discovery was that *cultured organisms could be attenuated.* In 1869 Moritz and others had ascertained the parasitic character of so-called chicken cholera, a destructive disease among fowls. Pasteur succeeded in attaining pure sub-cultures of the organism of this disease in chicken broth. He ascertained that infection was contained in the fowl's excreta and was spread by food. He also found that guinea pigs into which was inoculated fluid from a liquid culture of the chicken cholera microbe developed a relatively innocent local abscess, but otherwise remained well, unlike rabbits and fowls in similar circumstances. These observations of Pasteur are instructive even now. What could have been more natural than to regard the disease in fowls as originating spontaneously, although they acquired it when placed in the company of such inoculated guinea pigs? And yet the guinea pigs were responsible for the infection. "Let us throw away theories that we can disprove with convincing facts, but not on the vain pretext that some of their applications are incomprehensible."

On returning from his summer vacation in 1879, Pasteur was surprised to find that most of the cultures of fowl cholera left behind in his laboratory were no longer able to produce disease when inoculated into fowls. The virulence of the cultures had disappeared. But before abandoning the "spoilt" cultures Pasteur tested whether their inoculation into chickens produced any changes in them. He subsequently reinoculated these chickens with a new and powerful culture, without making them ill, while an identical inoculation was fatal to chickens obtained fresh from the market as a control.

Evidently Pasteur had *lighted on a method of vaccination.* It more nearly resembled the old inoculation of small pox from a mild case of this disease, than vaccination by cowpox; and it differed further that the virus of vaccinia and of variola are both unknown, while Pasteur was working with an identified organism.

How had this production of an attenuated vaccinal virus been obtained? Pasteur found experimentally that by prolonging the intervals of implantation in successive culture media, virulence was gradually attenuated, a milder disease developing—but more rapidly—in the inoculated fowl. He found, furthermore, that by protecting cultures brought to different degrees of attenuation he could maintain their virulence at this point when passed from culture to culture.

Emile Roux expressed the result thus: "Attenuation is hereditary. These viruses can be modified by culture like the higher plants. Pasteur has obtained varieties of virus as a gardener raises varieties of flowers."

Pasteur also observed that sometimes fowl cholera instead of killing produced a semi-chronic disease, and that the microbe obtained from these fowls had an increased virulence. Such a fact has obvious significance as an illustration of nature's procedure in preserving the microbes of a disease from annihilation, and it has a bearing on the "carrier" problem which has been elucidated in recent years (page 100).

The same facts were regarded by Pasteur as throwing light on the "possibility of prolonged incubations of a virus such, for example, as rabies;" and it is likely that at this early stage of his work Pasteur was already considering the possibility of attacking the problem of rabies.

The above experimental results were the background of Pasteur's investigation of anti-anthrax vaccination.

In June, 1880, W. S. Greenfield had shown that anthrax germs can be attenuated, i.e., reduced in virulence by culture in bovine aqueous humors; and in 1883 Pasteur definitely introduced his method of vaccination against this disease.

He had made his first experiments on anthrax in 1877 in collaboration with Joubert. He confirmed the presence and rapid multiplication of the long tangled filaments described by Koch in sterilized neutral urine. He diluted their growth by subculture of drops through a hundred generations and by similar reasoning to that of Koch concluded that anthrax is purely "the disease of the bacteridium, as trichinosis is the disease of the trichina, and scabies the disease of the acarus."

Pasteur found that the anthrax bacillus only developes with difficulty in cultures at temperatures of 43° to 44°C., and suggested that this might explain the natural immunity of the fowl to anthrax, as its normal temperature is 42°C. In confirmation of this he found the immunity of fowls disappeared, when by keeping their legs and lower body in water at 25°C. their body temperature was lowered to 37° to 38°C. which is the temperature of animals that are susceptible to anthrax. He also found that a fowl inoculated with anthrax was at once cured, if removed from the cold water as soon as the first symptoms of anthrax had appeared.

There followed the experimental investigation of anthrax in sheep by Pasteur's colleagues, P. W. Chamberland and Roux in the field. First spontaneous anthrax was investigated. Sheep were fed with lucerne watered with cultures of anthrax bacilli. Some died, others recovered. Eight of the latter were inoculated with cultures of anthrax or anthrax blood. All were ill, only one died. These results suggested a method of vaccination, and laboratory experiments were begun to this end. Virulent cultures of anthrax bacilli in broth were incubated at 42° to 43°C. At this temperature the power of producing spores had disappeared, and the virulence of the bacilli was lowered. After 12 days at this temperature the culture would not kill adult guinea pigs, and after 28 days longer it was harmless even to young mice and guinea pigs. Sporulation was allowed, and cultures sown with these spores reproduced an attenuated variety of anthrax bacilli. Thus were secured "virus vaccines fixed as spores with their particular characteristics, which can be transported without possibility of change."

The details of the subsequent successful vaccinations of sheep on a large scale need not be given, but that protection against anthrax was secured is without doubt. Later it appears that trouble arose over impure cultures, which is readily understood, as Pasteur did not employ Koch's newer methods of obtaining pure cultures, already available. But that by Pasteur's inoculations immense losses of cattle and sheep were avoided is clear. In later years this method of vaccination has been the means of saving vast herds in the Argentine. In England it has been employed but little, for it has been found that the disease can be controlled by a rigid system of notification of all cases and the destruction of infected carcases and of all contaminated matters. Given such measures the *champs maudits* cease to exist.

At a later date Pfeiffer and Neufeld have maintained that vaccines of killed bacilli may be substituted for the bacilli used by Pasteur which had been attenuated by groupng at temperatures higher than the body temperature; but whether this is so for anthrax or for fowl cholera is regarded by Ledingham as doubtful.

# CHAPTER VII

## The Prevention of Rabies

In the fertile mind of Pasteur his investigations of chicken cholera and anthrax appear to have suggested the possibility of specific prophylaxis against rabies. Why against a relatively rare disease like rabies rather than against such commonly fatal diseases as measles or tuberculosis? Rabies was only an occasional cause of death in France. In England since civil registration of deaths began in 1837, it has seldom caused more than 30 human deaths in any single year. The greatest number was 60 in 1883 (fig. 3) while the deaths from the two diseases named above numbered many thousands each year. But in Pasteur there was a flair for tasks approaching the impossible, and circumstances drew him to this particular problem; furthermore he was hot on the track of specific prophylaxis. He had been able to attenuate the virus of chicken cholera to an extent which meant only slight illness from it, and yet would protect a fowl against subsequent inoculation of a more virulent strain of virus.

In 1881 he had experimented with the virus (used here as synonymous for microbe, or microörganism) of anthrax, which previously had been attenuated to an extent rendering it incompetent to kill a guinea pig a few days old. He inoculated the first of a

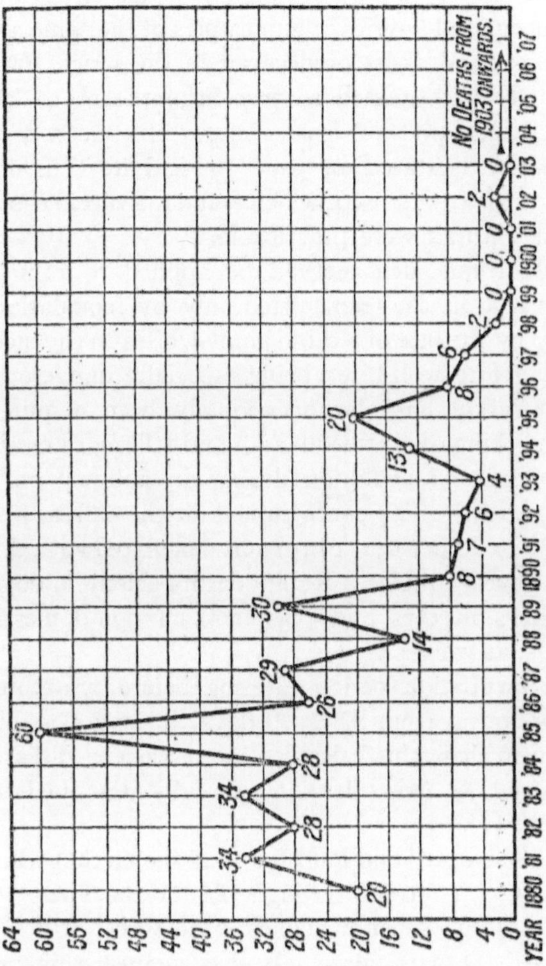


FIG. 3. ENGLAND AND WALES.—ANNUAL DEATHS FROM HYDROPHOBIA, 1880 TO 1902

series of one day old guinea pigs with this virus; and then inoculated a series of guinea pigs of the same age with the blood of its predecessor in the series, until eventually he obtained a virus incompetent to kill adult guinea pigs or even sheep. His method of attenuation is stated on page 50; and he thus obtained a *virus fixe*, with which standard vaccinations against anthrax were practicable.

Could some such method be applied to rabies? Rabies is a disease transmitted only by inoculation, usually by the bite of a rabid animal, bites on the face, and therefore wolf bites, being especially dangerous. The infection has also occasionally been acquired by the licking of a rabic animal, and still more rarely by accidental inoculation during an autopsy on a rabic patient. The contagium is in the saliva, and from 20 to 70 per cent of persons inoculated with this saliva develop rabies. Rabies occurs chiefly in dogs, sometimes in cats and pigs; also in non-domestic animals, as wolves or deer.

The incubation period elapsing before symptoms develop varies from 20 to 60 days; it may possibly be longer than this. Rabies is an ancient disease, mentioned by Aristotle. It was fully described by Mead in 1767.

In 1880 Nocard and Paul Bert had shown that when rabic saliva is filtered through plaster the virus remains on this substance; hence the virus, still unidentified, is particulate. It was against this unrecognised virus that Pasteur's investigation was directed. In this investigation, shared by Roux, Chamberland and Thullier, it was shown that the virus is in the nervous system of the affected animal as well as in its saliva; and at an early stage (in 1881) these investigators proved that rabies could easily be conveyed by trephining the skull and inoculating the rabic material under the dura mater.

Following the lines of Pasteur's earlier work on chicken cholera and anthrax, experiments were made with this unknown virus present in cerebral tissues, with a view to attenuate it. The virus was found to be increased in potency by passing through a series of rabbits, but attenuated at the end of a series of inoculations into monkeys.

But even if an attenuated virus were obtainable, was it wise to vaccinate before being bitten by a mad dog? This implied an incommoding experiment—at the best—to avoid the millionth chance of subsequently becoming rabic. At this point it appeared that either one must assume to be erroneous the accepted doctrine of inaccessibility of a virus once it has entered the human body, or one must abandon an unacceptable before-the-bite vaccination. Experimental proof was needed as to whether inoculation after infection has been acquired can be prophylactic.

Pasteur found that the increased virulence produced by passing the rabic virus from dog to rabbit and then through a series of rabbits, is associated with a diminished period of incubation, this becoming as short as seven days; also that when the virulence is diminished by passing the virus through monkeys, the reduced virulence persists when a dog is inoculated with this virus. He expressed his confidence in the possibility of after-the-bite vaccination as follows in 1884: "thanks to the length of time of incubation of rabies following bites, I have every reason to believe a refractory state may be established in those who have been bitten, before a mortal disease declares itself"; and that this was so, he subsequently demonstrated experimentally.

But the use of monkeys was impracticable on a considerable scale, and Pasteur then attempted to utilize exposure to oxygen, as in his experiments on anthrax and chicken cholera, to produce attenuation. Having prepared an intensive virus in rabbits with a minimum period of incubation, he suspended spinal cords from these animals in a dry air at 20°C. under careful precautions against contamination, and found that, thus treated, the virulence gradually decreased and disappeared, the time required for this varying with the thickness of the cord and the temperature of the air. He was now ready to attempt to immunize a dog against rabies.

An emulsion was made from one of the cords which had been longest submitted to this process of drying in dry air, and this was injected into a dog subcutaneously. On subsequent days a similar injection was made from cords which had been exposed a shorter time to air, until finally an emulsion from a virulent cord which had been exposed only 1 to 2 days was thus injected. Then came the crucial test. Virulent rabic material was introduced under the experimental dog's dura mater and the dog proved refractory to the disease. Many repetitions of the experiment proved the efficacy of this method, including its application after previous rabic inoculation.

News of the process soon spread and Pasteur was inundated with applications for the treatment of human beings bitten by rabic dogs or wolves; and finally after much hesitation he vaccinated Joseph Meister, a boy aged 9 years, who had lacerated wounds on hands and legs produced by a mad dog on the 4th of July. Beginning inoculations on the 6th of July with an emulsion derived from the cord of a rabic rabbit kept 15 days in a flask in dry air, injections from more recently dried cords were made each day, check experiments on rabbits being conducted throughout; and finally an injection was given which in the absence of the previous injections would have produced rabies. The boy remained well.

In accordance with Pasteur's method or methods modified from his, the practice of anti-rabic vaccination has become adopted in many countries. Of the first 350 patients thus treated by Pasteur, only one died, and this was a person in whom 37 days had elapsed since he was bitten and before the treatment was begun.

Between 1886 and 1905 over 15,000 persons had been inoculated, and the fatality among those thus treated was always less than 1 per cent and in years subsequent to 1887 varied between 0.55 and 0.18 per cent, a very small proportion when compared with the incidence of rabies in unvaccinated persons who had been bitten.

In some countries, as in some American States in which rabies is common, prophylactic vaccination of dogs has been made compulsory; and where the British method of control described in the next paragraph is impracticable, this appears desirable. It may be hoped, however, that this measure will eventually be unnecessary, and that Pasteurian vaccination will then be reserved for persons bitten by suspected dogs. Even in these cases it is important that the actual existence of rabies in the biting animals should be tested on rabbits in a satisfactory state laboratory.

Pasteur in writing to Sir James Paget in London in August, 1886, had suggested the desirability of the British Government authorizing him to vaccinate all the dogs in the Isle of Mauritius—in which rabies was common,—and that after securing the surveillance of all dogs subsequently coming into the island, there would then be provided a large scale test of the efficacy of his method of vaccination.

But Great Britian was fated to be the island in which this demonstration was successfully made. In figure 3 is shown the number of human deaths from rabies annually registered in England and Wales from 1880 to 1902, after which year no human deaths from this disease have occurred. Mr. Walter (afterwards Lord) Long in 1896, on behalf of the British Government enacted a Muzzling Order for the whole country, which was rigidly enforced during that year; and at the same time was begun the system of not allowing any dog to be introduced from over-seas except after six months' quarantine. The regulations were continued notwithstanding much agitation from the selfishly tender-hearted owners of pet dogs; and rabies from that time became extinct both in man and animals, except for an accidental group of cases in dogs during the Great War, due to a failure in administration. The action taken demonstrated that at the present time rabies only occurs when acquired from another rabic animal, and that it can be completely controlled by administrative measures.

# CHAPTER VIII

## The Prevention of Diphtheria

The discoveries briefly described in the three last chapters showed the possibility of preventing attack from three diseases,—chicken cholera, anthrax, and rabies,—by prophylactic vaccination. In the case of diphtheria, and of a few other diseases further triumphs over infection have been secured. In diphtheria the first success was in ensuring marvellous mitigation of an already developed attack of the disease by serum therapeutics; but more recently increased knowledge of bacteriology has led to the discovery of successful prophylactic inoculation.

The seriousness of diphtheria as a cause of national mortality can be seen from the following table, relating to England. In continental countries it is an

*England and Wales. Annual death rates per million of population*

| | Maximum | Minimum |
|---|---|---|
| Diphtheria | 318 in 1893 | 93 in 1872 |
| Scarlet fever | 1,054 in 1874 | 22 in 1917 |
| Small pox | 1,012 in 1871 | 0 in seven years (1911–1920) |
| Measles | 602 in 1887 | 96 in 1919 |
| Whooping cough | 710 in 1878 | 71 in 1919 |
| Typhus | 121 in 1871 | 0 in 1911–1920 |
| Enteric fever | 377 in 1872 | 14 in 1920 |

even greater cause of death. For convenience I give the maximum and minimum death rates between 1871

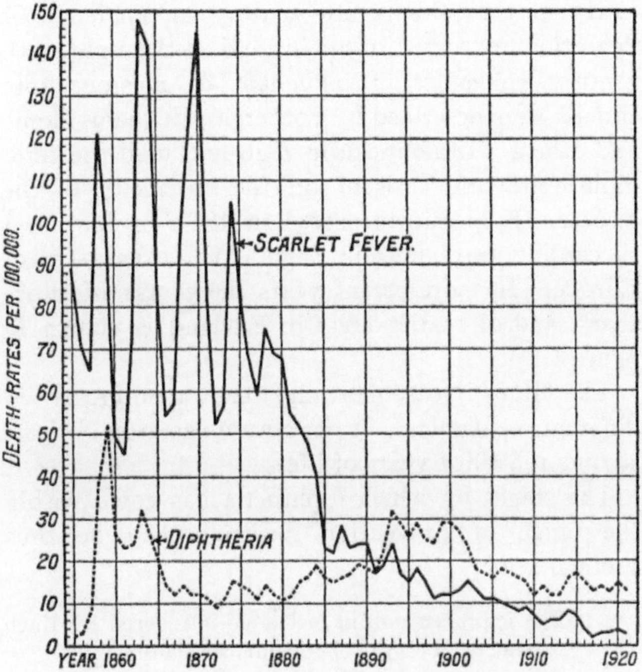


FIG. 4. ANNUAL DEATH-RATES FROM DIPHTHERIA AND SCARLET FEVER, ENGLAND AND WALES

and 1921 for diphtheria and a number of other acute infectious diseases.

Diphtheria has been recognised for ages. Hippocrates probably alluded to it in describing a "web on the tonsil," and in medieval writings are many references to a suffocative disease of the throat. Early in the seventeenth century an epidemic of "garotillo" occurred in Spain; and in the eighteenth century epidemics of malignant or ulcerous sore throats were described by Fothergill, Huxham, Home and others. Bretonneau in 1826 first used the term diphthérite and insisted on the specificity of the disease. Epidemics occurred in 1849, in 1857 and succeeding years, both in England and other parts of Europe. In more recent years the course of diphtheria and of scarlet fever in England is shown in figure 4.

The fatality (case mortality) has varied greatly in different epidemics. It is always greatest in the second and third years of life.

The stages by which diphtheria has come within the range of preventive medicine may be thus summarised.

1. The improvements in technique introduced by Koch rendered it easy to obtain unmixed cultures.
2. Weigert's introduction of aniline dyes in 1874 rendered the detection of the diphtheria bacillus easy.
3. In 1883 Klebs identified the bacillus, and in 1884 Löffler proved its causal relation to diphtheria. Hence the name commonly employed—Klebs-Löffler bacillus.
4. The bacilli it was found were strictly limited to the site of the local lesions.

How then was the terribly lethal effect of the disease in children produced? Löffler suggested that a toxin was formed, and that this toxin would be present in the bouillon in which Klebs-Löffler bacilli were cultivated.

In 1887 Roux and Yersin in Pasteur's laboratory set themselves to work out this problem. With them—and the same might be said of nearly all of Pasteur's work,—it was a humanitarian crusade even more than a scientific investigation. The bacilli found in the throats of children suffering from diphtheria were grown in flasks of broth, and animals were inoculated with the growth. Rabbits thus treated developed paralysis of their limbs, just as children did in clinical diphtheria; and as in children, apart from the naso-pharnyx, no bacilli were found in the rabbits' tissues.

Roux and Yersin then filtered the inseminated bouillon containing a four day old growth of diphtheria bacilli through porcelain candles under high pressure, thus securing a clear germless fluid. Peritoneal injections of this fluid into guinea pigs produced no effect, until enormous quantities were given. Evidently there was no toxin or the toxin was very feeble. But when the inseminated culture of diphtheria bacilli was kept before filtration for 42 days instead of 4 and then injected into guinea pigs, paralysis was at once produced, thus showing the slow formation of the toxin.

Almost simultaneously, working in Koch's laboratory, E. L. Behring was making similar experiments. He took some guinea pigs which had survived the illness following earlier injections of Klebs-Löffler bacilli, and found that they remained well in spite of further gigantic doses of these bacilli. They had become immune. Then blood was abstracted from these guinea pigs, left to clot, and the serum collected. Behring next, as Roux had done, injected the filtrate from a bouillon growth of bacilli into some of these recovered guinea pigs. They were unaffected. In short such guinea pigs were immune against large doses of powerful diphtheria toxin.

Next came the final test. Serum from a guinea pig recovered after an attack of diphtheria was added in a glass tube to an active virulent broth culture of Klebs-Löffler bacilli. This mixture was inoculated into a new non-immune guinea pig, *but no attack was produced.* Check experiments with serum from a healthy non-immune guinea pig gave no inhibition of disease. Plainly then *the serum of immune animals was curative.* It destroyed or neutralised the toxin of diphtheria: hence its name antitoxin.

In 1891 the first child, who was desperately ill with diphtheria in a Berlin hospital, was treated with this antitoxin with a favorable result.

Roux was mainly instrumental in bringing the subject from the experimental to the practical stage. He discovered an easy method to make horses immune, and thus was able to obtain large quantities of antitoxin. In reporting his results to the International Congress of Hygiene at Buda Pesth in 1894, to an enthusiastic audience including the present writer, Roux was able to announce that the fatality from diphtheria in the Paris Children's Hospital had already been reduced from 52 to 25 per cent in children suffering from diphtheria.

Since then the value of antitoxin in diphtheria has been abundantly proved, though statistics showing this have been traversed. A larger proportion of the total cases of diphtheria are recognised, since diagnosis of doubtful cases by examination of secretions from the throat in doubtful sore throat has been practised, and the type of diphtheria may vary from time to time; but after full allowance for these and like causes of variation, there has been a vast saving of life by the antitoxin treatment of diphtheria; and as saving of life by improved treatment forms an important branch of preventive medicine, the discovery of antitoxin must rank as marking a great advance.

The most impressive lines of evidence of life-saving by antitoxin consist (1) in the reduction of proportion of total cases of diphtheria requiring tracheotomy; (2) in the reduction in fatality (case mortality) of tracheotomy cases; and (3) in the evidence that the curative effect of antitoxin is greater in proportion with the promptness of its administration.

Two illustrations may be given from experience in the London Fever Hospitals (1900–1909).

| | Per cent fatality |
|---|---|
| Laryngeal cases: | |
| *a.* 7,445 cases treated with antitoxin | 18.3 |
| *b.* 129 cases not treated with antitoxin | 57.2 |
| Cases needing tracheotomy: | |
| *a.* 3,128 cases treated with antitoxin | 30.8 |
| *b.* 59 cases not treated with antitoxin | 86.5 |

Evidently if antitoxin has no value as a remedy, the day of its administration is immaterial; but the experiences of some 20,000 cases in various experiences in several countries gave the following results:

Among the cases treated by antitoxin the fatality (case mortality) varied as follows:

| | per cent |
|---|---|
| On the 1st day of disease | 2.2– .86 |
| On the 2nd day of disease | 6.6– 8.3 |
| On the 3rd day of disease | 8.6–17.1 |
| On the 4th day of disease | 17.0–25.5 |
| On the 5th day of disease | 23.2–35.3 |

It can thus be stated that the results of clinical experience confirm those derived from exact scientific experimentation on animals.

In discussing diphtheria in relation to the administration of antitoxin it is necessary to distinguish between case mortality (fatality) and incidence in the total population as shown by the number of cases or deaths from diphtheria in that population. The fatality of attacked persons may be reduced by antitoxin while an epidemic of diphtheria is increasing, for antitoxin does not prevent a case of diphtheria from being infectious. The causes of epidemicity of diphtheria are imperfectly known; but as seen in figure 4 it becomes a serious epidemic disease at uncertain intervals, and generally is much more prevalent in the cities of continental countries such as America, France and Germany than in the cities of England. There is some obscure relationship between these epidemics and pandemics and a succession of years with exceptionally low rainfall. In New York, in which most valuable work has been done in immunizing the young against diphtheria, the lowest death-rate in terms of population, that of 1924, was as high as that of London in which little artificial immunization has hitherto been secured.

Before leaving the question of administration of antitoxin, attention should be drawn to the failure often experienced to give antitoxin promptly in an attack of diphtheria. Dr. Caiger writing in 1923 on the basis of experience in hospitals in London stated that 30 per cent of the fatal cases died within 24 hours of admission to hospital. Some of this delay in admission to hospital and in treatment by antitoxin may have been the result of waiting for bacteriological confirmation of the diagnosis, which is unjustifiable in diphtheria. The facts display that in a considerable proportion of cases shiftless or indifferent parents or dilatory doctors are responsible for much of the mortality from diphtheria.

The discovery of antitoxin for diphtheria was a triumph of laboratory research, the outcome of experimental work on immunity; the progress of this research can be seen from stage to stage, and it constitutes an epochal point in the history of medicine.

In 1913 Von Behring suggested a new method for actively immunizing against attack by diphtheria by means of diphtheria toxin-antitoxin.

In the same year Dr. Béla Schick demonstrated that the intracutaneous injection of one-fiftieth of a lethal dose of the toxin of diphtheria per 254 grams of weight of guinea pig sufficed to produce a specific local inflammation—white urticarial wheals—in an individual who has no antitoxic substances in his system. This reaction fails if at least one thousandth of an antitoxic unit is present in 1 cubic centimeter of the blood serving the tested individual (Schick's Harvey Lecture, 1922–1923). On the other hand, if the individual is naturally immune the antitoxin circulating in his blood neutralises the toxin injected into his skin, and no skin reaction appears. It has been found that some 50 per cent of children under the age of 10 respond to the test, the proportion then gradually decreasing.

It appears clear that many persons receive a dosage of diphtheria infection which does not suffice to produce a clinical attack, but is adequate to develop enough antitoxin-toxin to prevent such an attack.

By Schick's test it is possible to distinguish persons liable to be attacked by diphtheria and to immunize or otherwise protect these, while ignoring others whose Schick reaction is negative. Children from six months to seven years old are specially menaced; in later years of life it can be demonstrated that an increasing amount of antitoxin is present in the blood serum. In the early months of infancy protective substances are also present. In the blood of the umbilical cord Fischl and Wunscheim have shown this to be so in 80 per cent of the cases examined.

Active immunity against diphtheria is obtained by administering a mixture of toxin and antitoxin. The toxin used in the Schick test requires to be carefully standardized, and so does the mixed toxin and antitoxin for producing active immunity. The method of immunization thus rendered available has been used on a large scale in New York by Park and Zingher. Over two million children in New York State and large numbers in other parts of America, as well as smaller numbers elsewhere have been thus immunized.

More recently diphtheria toxin has been treated with formalin, and its toxicity thus reduced: and it would appear that this use of toxoid and toxoid-antitoxin gives good results without some of the disadvantages of the earlier method. A series of injections are given, occupying a period of two or three weeks. Immunity does not immediately develop, but is increasingly established in 3 to 9 months. It would appear that the active immunity thus developed is comparable with the immunization established as adult life is approached by most members of an urban community; presumably by intermittent exposure to small doses of infective material, inadequate to cause a definite clinical attack. The evidence so far gathered points to effective protection lasting for at least six years, which means artificial protection at the most dangerous ages, this protection merging into the natural acquired immunity of adult life. The method has also proved its value in protecting nurses exposed to diphtheria infection; and it can be applied with great success to susceptible children in residential institutions when an outbreak of diphtheria occurs.

It is too early as yet to give complete statistical proof of the protection afforded a community against diphtheria by general immunization of children by toxin-antitoxin. The unknown factors of epidemicity may break through local defenses in future years, if active immunization has not been universal, or if its effect has worn out with time. Persons giving a negative Schick reaction may themselves be "carriers" of Klebs-Löffler bacilli. But the triple armamentarium of antitoxin, of the Schick test of immunity, and the giving of toxin-antitoxin to confer immunity on susceptible persons, especially children and attendants on the sick has placed diphtheria in the front rank as a preventible disease; and already, subject to the considerations noted above, the diminution of diphtheria has been very marked in some American communities, following on the extensive immunization of local populations. Thus in New Haven, Connecticut, the death rate from diphtheria in 1924 was 1.7 per 10,000 population as compared with 11.2 for the whole of Connecticut. In some townships in the State of New York after successful propaganda and inoculations, diphtheria has been at least temporarily wiped out of clinical existence.

# CHAPTER IX

## Bacteriology in Relation to Immunity and to Diagnosis

The most striking phenomenon in an attack of an infectious disease is its effect in preventing recurrence after recovery. Erysipelas, pneumonia, and influenza are partial or entire exceptions to this statement; but in measles, small pox, whooping cough and some others a second attack, when exposure to infection occurs is rare. In diphtheria and scarlet fever the immunity conferred by one attack, is less certain; a second attack of syphilis occurs rarely; two or three attacks of typhus are not unknown.

Even for the same disease there appears to be evidence that members of certain families incur greater risks than others of acquiring diphtheria or scarlet fever or typhoid fever when exposed to them, though this difference is rarely very marked.

Our knowledge of means for producing immunity which is not natural or innate, and is not the result of an attack of the disease in question, has rapidly increased. There was a long interval between the publication of Jenner's famous Inquiry in 1798 and further developments. These had to wait for Pasteur who was much influenced by Jenner's discovery of vaccination against small pox. In Chapters VI to VIII an account of Pasteur's work in discovering methods of vaccination against chicken cholera, anthrax and rabies has been given.

Theories as to the mechanism of protection have varied. The two chief theories for some years were that of exhaustion of the pabulum required by the microbe for its continued multiplication, and the retention theory of Chauveau, which assumed that further multiplication of the microbe was inhibited by the accumulation of the products of bacterial activity.

In 1884 Metschnikoff (1845—1916) observed that in water fleas the wandering cells of the body surrounded and gradually absorbed into their substance particles of pigment or yeast cells swallowed by the flea. On these and similar experiments he based his theory of phagocytosis, as responsible for securing immunity against infection. It soon became evident that, while body cells were active in the production of immunity, other factors were involved, and much controversy arose between those who regarded the cells of the body and those who thought that the blood serum was responsible for immunity. Later on some reconciliation between the two views became possible, when the discoveries of Denys, Wright and others showed that certain substances in the blood serum prepare invading microörganisms for phagocytosis by the leucocytes.

Nuttall in 1888 advanced our knowledge of the anti-bacterial properties of the body fluids, especially of blood serum; and this work was followed by that of

Pfeiffer, who in 1894 showed that cholera spirilla introduced into the peritoneal cavity of immunized guinea pigs, or introduced with immune serum into the peritoneal cavity of normal guinea pigs lose their motility and break up into small granules. This is known as "Pfeiffer's phenomenon." It showed that a specific substance is present in immune serum which is concerned in the bacteriolytic process.

In 1890 Behring had already ascertained the protective and curative value of antitoxic serum (page 64). In 1896 the Pfeiffer phenomenon was demonstrated for the typhoid bacillus.

In 1895 while studying the conditions of the Pfeiffer phenomenon outside the body Bordet noted that when a small quantity of immune serum is added to a bouillon of cholera spirilla, these lose their motility and become agglutinated. Durham in 1896 published the result of a systematic study of the agglutinating and immobilising properties of immune serum from cases of enteric fever outside the body; and a little later in the same year Widal took the next step by showing that the agglutinating reaction takes place during an attack of enteric fever. Durham had already shown the importance of diluting the serum by which means it was possible to diagnose for instance between serum from cases of enteric fever and serum taken from patients suffering from invasion by the *Bac. enteritidis* of Gaertner.

Thus while investigating the general problem of immunity there had been discovered a method of serum diagnosis, by which several infectious diseases can be differentiated.

A further instance of blood reactions as a test for disease is that of the Wassermann reaction (page 170).

The following are the chief instances in which an artificial immunity against disease by means of laboratory products has been attempted with more or less success.

In 1890 Von Behring with Kitasato showed that the blood serum of an animal previously immunised against tetanus when injected into other animals protected these against poisoning with tetanus toxin, and against infection with living tetanus bacilli. This discovery was applied with marked success in the Great War, 1914–1918. In veterinary practice, in which it can be employed under test conditions, it appears to be an infallible protective against the effects of contamination by tetanus bacilli from the soil.

In 1888 Garmaleia succeeded in protecting guinea pigs and pigeons against infection with an organism *Vibrio Metschnikovi* by the previous inoculation of killed cultures of this organism.

Haffkine showed that inoculation of dead cultures of cholera spirilla led to the appearance of specific anti-bacterial substances in the blood serum and to the protection of the individual.

Following on these earlier observations there was great activity in testing dead bacilli. A. E. Wright (*Lancet*, September, 1896) published a note on a method of protecting against enteric fever by dead cultures, and Pfeiffer and Kolle independently (November, 1896) described a similar procedure. In this year a number of volunteers were vaccinated according to both these methods.

During the Boer War in 1899 voluntary inoculations on Wright's plan were given on a considerable scale. The results were obscured by failure to recognise the paratyphoid group of infections, against which inoculation by unmixed dead typhoid cultures was inert. The experience of the British garrison during the siege of Ladysmith is, however, suggestive.

| | Number in group | Cases of enteric fever |
|---|---|---|
| Uninoculated | 10,529 | 1,489 |
| Inoculated | 1,705 | 35 |

The antigenic properties of Wright's vaccine were later improved by reducing the temperature used in sterilization to 53°C.

In the Great War mixed cultures of typhoid and paratyphoid bacilli were used in inoculation, after killing the bacilli. The details of the results obtained can be studied in Leishman's account in the Official History of the War.

American Army experience is particularly useful as it relates to inoculation in circumstances in which other sanitary reforms were almost inoperative. In 1908 during the war with Spain enteric fever caused great havoc. As compared with this may be given Major F. F. Russell's account of the compulsory inoculation of troops in the manœuvres on the Mexican frontier in 1911. There were on the borders three divisional camps, each camp in full occupation for four months.

| | Cases in troops | In civilian population |
|---|---|---|
| Galveston Camp (4,500 men)............... | None | 192 |
| San Diego (3,000 men)...................... | 2 | |
| San Antonio (13,000 men).................. | 2 | |

Although the exact figures in the civilian population cannot be given there can be no reasonable doubt of the protective influence of the anti-typhoid inoculations. The immunisation in the United States Army is repeated every three years.

Haffkine in 1897 introduced for anti-plague inoculation a broth culture of the *Bac. pestis* which had been sterilized by heating to 65°C., and this vaccine was employed with much success.

The methods of vaccination against chicken cholera, anthrax, and rabies have already been described.

In 1907 Theobald Smith first suggested that a toxin-antitoxin mixture might be used in immunisation, and in 1912 such a mixture was employed by Behring. In 1913 Schick reported his cutaneous toxin reaction for determining immunity from diphtheria, and thus a toxin-antitoxin mixture to protect against diphtheria could be given with scientific exactitude.

More recently a similar test of susceptibility (the Dick test) has been introduced for scarlet fever, and for this disease there is good evidence that the inoculation of blood serum derived from a case convalescent from it modifies and curtails an attack of scarlet fever. In measles the use of serum from patients recovered from measles has also been employed with encouraging success.

These more recent advances in diagnosis, in immunisation and in treatment will doubtless be extended and improved.

The question naturally arises whether by some of the preceding methods a more general protection of the population and especially of children against infectious diseases may be expected. The advances already made give much ground for hope.

Small pox and diphtheria already are within the range of practicable complete prevention by vaccination. If measles and whooping cough could be brought within the same category, it would be an immense boon; for these two diseases are not only responsible for a very heavy loss of young life, but they also leave behind them disabling deafness or other weaknesses and are a great cause of national ill-health. Immunisation against enteric fever and all ingested infections stands in a different position. In well governed communities sanitary administration can control them and anti-typhoid or allied vaccinations are indicated mainly in exceptional circumstances (page 119).

Various attempts have been made to immunise against catarrhs, with doubtful and erratic success. The whole group of catarrhal infections forms a wide barren patch in the field of preventive medicine. Bronchitis, even in the absence of provocative dusty occupations is a wide-spread disease. Pneumonia although three types of pneumococcus have been identified, and one of them is favourably affected by serum treatment, still is a chief cause of death. Cerebrospinal fever sometimes is favourably influenced by anti-meningococcic serum, but our chief reliance in this disease is in general hygiene. Against poliomyelitis and the still more serious disease epidemic encephalitis we have, hitherto, no defence

Tuberculosis is another disease in which hope of a curative tuberculin or of a specific prophylactic have hitherto been grievously disappointed. But here again it is clear that personal and public hygiene—if adequately pursued by all—suffices to secure a much more rapid decline than is at present being realised.

The name of Paul Ehrlich (1854–1915) is associated with the most brilliant work in immunology and in chemo-therapeutics. His "side-chain" theory, however fantastic, has proved very valuable in developing the science of immunity and of serum reactions. He assumed that a molecule of protoplasm contains a stable nucleus and unstable side-chains (chemo-receptors) which can combine with food substances and neutralize toxins by detaching side-chains into the blood. Having found that protozoal diseases could not be treated by special antitoxins he tried various chemical agents, particularly for syphilis, which after many failures resulted in the discovery of 606. In founding this new branch of preventive medicine Ehrlich's name deserves to stand with those of Pasteur and Koch, who had laid the foundations of general bacteriology.

# CHAPTER X

## The Prevention of Cholera

We come next to the consideration of infectious diseases, the control of which has been secured in the main apart from any attempt to confer artificial immunity against them. In this respect they resemble sepsis, the almost complete abolition of which has been secured in the practice of surgery.

As seen in Chapter XVII of *Evolution of Preventive Medicine*, the home of cholera is in India, from which it has at intervals invaded Europe and America, sometimes with devastating results. The annual number of recorded deaths from cholera in India during a series of years is shown in figure 5. Without repeating what appears in the above named chapter, the following particulars may be given.

Cholera is a disease in the prevention of which the object is to prevent access of the infecting agent to the alimentary canal of a human being. It belongs in this respect to the same group as enteric fever and dysentery. In all three, without direct attack on the infecting agent in the body, it suffices to stop an epidemic if we break the link of infection, which is carried in some ingested matter. Whatever be the unknown factors which eventuate in cholera undertaking, so to speak, its maleficent travels westward over the world, we know that all links of infection can be broken by the effective method of intervention noted above, quite as successfully as an entire community can be thrown into darkness by making a breach of continuity in its electric light main.

Cholera, when prevalent on a large scale, is usually transmitted by a contaminated water supply. The first pandemic of modern times occurred in 1817–

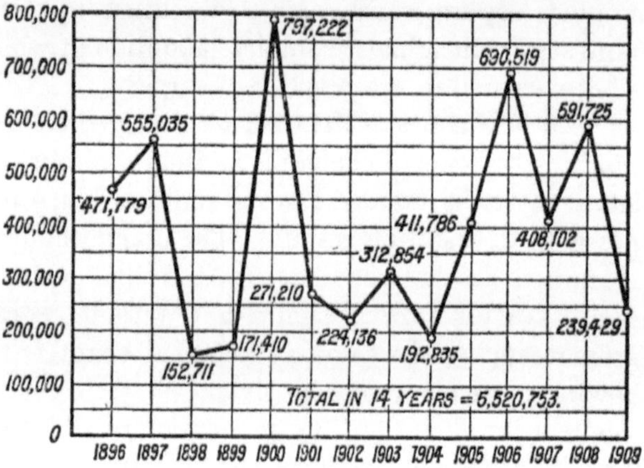


FIG. 5

1823: it only reached the frontiers of Europe. The second, in 1826–1837 reached Germany through Russia by three routes and was brought to England at Sunderland by a boat from Hamburg. It spread slowly through the winter, and in June, 1832, was carried to Canada by Irish emigrants, reaching the United States about the same time. It died out in the winter of 1837–1838.

The third pandemic began in 1846, and with a lull in 1850–1852 lasted till 1863. It reached North America in 1848, and spread over the entire northern hemisphere. The fourth pandemic of 1865–1875 was brought to England in 1865 in a ship from Alexandria to Southampton. In May, 1866, it was brought from Rotterdam to Liverpool, and other invasions followed. In 1866 it attacked Halifax in Nova Scotia, and New York and New Orleans were also implicated. Russia was a center of dissemination of infection throughout this pandemic.

In 1873 some further cases occurred in England, but there was no serious extension. So far as England and Wales are concerned, the toll on life in the chief epidemic years since registration of deaths began in 1837, can be seen from the following table:

| Year | England and Wales | | London | |
|---|---|---|---|---|
| | Deaths from cholera | Death rate per 10,000 | Deaths from cholera | Death rate per 10,000 |
| 1849 | 53,293 | 30 | 13,565 | 51 |
| 1854 | 20,097 | 11 | 10,684 | 43 |
| 1866 | 14,378 | 7 | 5,548 | 8 |

Von Pettenkofer (1818–1901) held the view that in the evolution of the contagium of cholera a part of its life history must be spent in the soil; and for many years his views received acceptance with hygienists. Although John Snow (1813–1858) had previously stated the true teaching as to spread by means of infected water, and had given an almost complete epidemiological demonstration of this, Simon in his report to the President of the General Board of Health in 1856 arrived at the conclusion that "under the specific influence which determines an epidemic period, fecalised drinking water and fecalised air equally may breed and carry the poison" (of cholera).

In his report to the Privy Council in 1866, Simon once more stated: "Here in Europe the pestilence rages only where there are definite sanitary evils. . . . . Excrement sodden earth, excrement reeking air, excrement tainted water, these are for us the causes of cholera." In the same report, while endorsing N. Radcliffe's conclusion as to the water origin of an outbreak in East London, Simon in view of some anomalies of local distribution of disease suggested that water may have "operated on or through the soil of the territory."

The most striking instance of the failure of Pettenkofer's localist hypothesis to explain outbreaks of cholera and a further illustration of the truth of Snow's induction is supplied by the experience of Hamburg and Altona in August 1892.

In August 128 fatal cases of cholera occurred in Hamburg before the 23rd of the month. Some delay occurred in regarding the cases as cholera, owing to difficulty in verifying the diagnosis by finding Koch's comma bacilli in the dejecta of patients. This illustrates, as has often been illustrated in diphtheria, the danger of postponing field investigation and action until the bacterial identity of a disease has been certified.

Hamburg is situated on the right bank of the tidal part of the river Elbe, with a population in 1892 which is given below. Its sewers discharged into the river just below the town, and its water supply was drawn from the river just above the town. This water was pumped directly into depositing tanks and thence into supply pipes without any treatment. Altona is a smaller town on the opposite side of the Elbe.

During the period August 12 to October 23 the number of cases of cholera was as follows:

| | Population | Cases of cholera | Case rate per 10,000 population |
|---|---|---|---|
| Hamburg | 640,000 | About 17,000 | 134 |
| Altona | 143,000 | About 500 | 22 |

Hamburg's water supply was from the Elbe above the city. Altona's supply was received from the Elbe at a point below where Hamburg's sewage entered into it, as well as the sewage of a considerable outside population; but there was an efficient system of filtration of the Altona supply of water through sand before its distribution. That the water supply constituted the crucial difference between the two communities of Hamburg and Altona was further shown by the special experience of certain groups of people. Thus there were 2075 persons in 4 institutions in Hamburg including two prisons, which were supplied with water from their own wells. Not a case of cholera occurred in them. Again there were two rows of dwelling houses on the Hamburg side of the boundary line between the two cities, comprising 72 separate tenements and 400 people. Owing to local difficulties Hamburg water could not conveniently be supplied to these, and Altona water had been laid on to them from a neighboring street. No cases of cholera occurred in them.

The filter beds for the Altona water were composed of sand and gravel. Koch's investigation showed that the immunity of Altona was due to the carefully regulated and slow process of filtration and to the layer of mud on the top of the sand which retained the solid matter in the water including bacteria. Whenever this surface layer was scraped off a great increase of microörganisms occurred in the effluent water.

In 1883 the comma bacillus of cholera was discovered by Koch in the contents and walls of the intestine of cholera patients; also in infected tanks in India. Although the disease is not inoculable in animals, the causal relation of this microbe to cholera is established. It has been the cause of cholera in laboratories during experimental work. No disease, except possibly plague, has caused so much panic among threatened or invaded people as cholera. The following instance taken from *Notes and Recollections of a Professional Life,* by Dr. W. Ferguson, 1846, is but one of many instances that might be cited:

When the Asiatic cholera prevailed, which is as much a contagion as the thunderstorm, disgraceful scenes occurred. Shipwrecked sailors were stoned upon the beach at K in Scotland under suspicion of coming from infected countries: wayfaring women, taken in labour were thrust from out houses where they had sheltered into the highways of Ayrshire.

Other media than water may convey the infection of either typhoid fever or cholera, the most important of these being milk contaminated by water, and oysters and other shell-fish derived from sewage contaminated layings. In fact, after most parts of England had become supplied with pure drinking water, little further reduction of enteric fever was secured until these additional sources of infection had been minimised, and until "carriers" of infections themselves not ill had been discovered and safeguarded against (page 98). Cholera may also be acquired in nursing a cholera patient in the absence of exact precautions. Personal infection in crowded slums increases its spread.

Quarantine regulations against its spread have never succeeded in countries having communication by land; and in England marine quarantine has been abandoned in favour of medical examination of all persons on an incoming vessel, detention of suspected patients, and surveillance at their home-destination of those arriving on vessels having had cholera patients on them.

## CHAPTER XI

### The Prevention of Enteric or Typhoid Fever

A short sketch of the early history of enteric (typhoid) fever was given in Chapters XV and XVI of *Evolution of Preventive Medicine*, with special reference to its differentiation from typhus fever. This differentiation was a necessary preliminary to accurate preventive measures. Such a differentiation as already indicated (page 23) does not imply a fixed dogma as to the permanence of each disease. In enteric fever several types of typhoid organisms associated with differing clinical syndromes have been identified; and for typhus fever also it may be that in Mexican typhus we have a persistent variant of typhus. The recent prevalence of variola minor in America and Western Europe, which appears to "breed true," also gives warning against too rigid views as to permanency of type of any particular disease. But it would be a serious injury to preventive medicine were such possible evolutionary variations in disease to divert attention from the organised preventive measures which are made possible by recognition of each disease and knowledge of its laws of origin and spread.

The more recent history of enteric fever is one of rapidly increasing control. Like cholera it is spread almost solely by ingestion of specifically contaminated food or drink, and like other diseases of the same group is especially controllable by sanitary measures, as will appear in the following pages.

In 1880 Eberth first detected the *Bacillus typhosus* in the spleen and mesenteric glands of a typhoid patient, and in 1884 Gaffky grew this organism in pure culture. In 1885 the *Bac. coli communis* was identified by Escherich, and then began discussion as to the possible evolution of the *B. typhosus* from this common intestinal organism in special circumstances. Hartley quotes Roux and Rodet as maintaining in 1890 that the two bacteria could not be distinguished. That this view was untenable became evident with the development of the serum tests described on page 74; and the same tests confirm the causal relation of the *Bac. typhosus* to the disease, although this cannot be demonstrated by animal inoculations except possibly in anthropoid apes. The results of anti-typhoid vaccinations (page 76) confirm this.

There is no proof that typhoid bacilli multiply outside the body, though they remain alive and are resistant to desiccation in the absence of sunlight.

Although protective vaccination against enteric fever is practicable, and in certain circumstances desirable (page 76) it is uncalled for in a general population where sanitary measures are practicable. Enteric fever historically has been reduced to a shadow of its past without the help of anti-typhoid vaccination; but in some circumstances, as during a war when unsanitary conditions may not be controllable, it is indicated. Civilian experience has shown that given notification of each known case in a given area to a responsible and competent health officer, given intensive study of all recognised casesand the detection of missing links of infection whether "carriers" or clinical cases, and given especially an investigation of possible infection from water or food, enteric fever can be rapidly brought under control.

The history of reduction of enteric fever in civilised countries is wrapped up with that of the growth of various branches of sanitary administration. Among these, first place belongs to reform in water supplies which is considered in a later paragraph.

The first demonstration of the origin of enteric fever from "contaminated water supply" appears to have been made at Lausen in Switzerland in 1872. Lausen was a village of 784 people, among whom enteric fever had previously been unknown. Its water supply was derived from a spring at the foot of a moraine gravel ridge 300 feet high lying between Lausen and the Fühler valley. In this valley one to two miles from Lausen was an isolated farm where lived a man who had recently returned from a distant visit. On June 10 he failed with enteric fever, and by the end of July three more cases occurred in the same house. The discharges from these patients were thrown into a brook, in which the farm's washing was also done. Between July 15 and the end of July this stream was dammed up to irrigate the meadows;

and it was noticed then, as on former occasions that the water in the Lausen spring had increased in amount. Experiments with sodium chloride proved connection between the stream and the spring, but flour was unable to penetrate. The outbreak among the Lausen villagers corresponded in time to this period of damming up the stream on the opposite side of the ridge.

In 1874 Buchanan described a localised outbreak of enteric fever in Caius College, Cambridge due to the insuction into water pipes of foecal matter during intermissions in the water service.

In 1879 at Caterham near London a wide-spread outbreak of enteric fever occurred in the area of its water supply. This was derived from a deep well and adits driven in the chalk strata. Within a fortnight 47 cases occurred in 35 houses in Caterham and 132 cases in 96 houses in Redhill, having water from the same source. There had been no previous cases for several years. Of the 47 first affected, 45 had drunk this water and 2 had frequented houses to which it was supplied. The incidence of the outbreak was similarly significant in the Redhill district. In the weeks preceding the outbreak extensions of the well were in progress, and it was proved that a man had worked in it who was suffering from a slight enteric attack, acquired in a neighboring town, and that he had eased himself below about a fortnight before the outbreak. It was estimated that during this fortnight 1,861,000 gallons of water had been pumped for the public supply, and that the water could not have contained more than a grain of excremental matter per gallon. The case illustrates the possibility that chemical analysis of a water may fail to detect pollution; and that there should be not only chemical and bacteriological examinations of water, but also rigid supervision of possibilities of contamination. Many other illustrations of cataclysmic epidemics of enteric fever from sudden contamination might be given. Two of these must suffice, both in English experience.

Maidstone (population 34,000) had an explosive outbreak of enteric fever in which 40 patients apparently had been infected prior to August 26, 1897 and 200 more developed symptoms between that date and September 12. Altogether some 800 cases occurred without including secondary cases in households. The time incidence of all the cases in a series of weeks is shown in figure 6.

Worthing (population 15,000) had a similar explosive outbreak, as shown also in figure 6. In this town 6.3 per cent and in Maidstone 5.3 per cent of the total population were attacked. In each place it will be noted that the outbreak culminated in the second week.

Each of the outbreaks was caused by accidental foecal contamination of the water supply, in Maidstone probably by vagrants, in Worthing by a workman working underground. Maidstone's water supply was derived from 18 springs, several of which

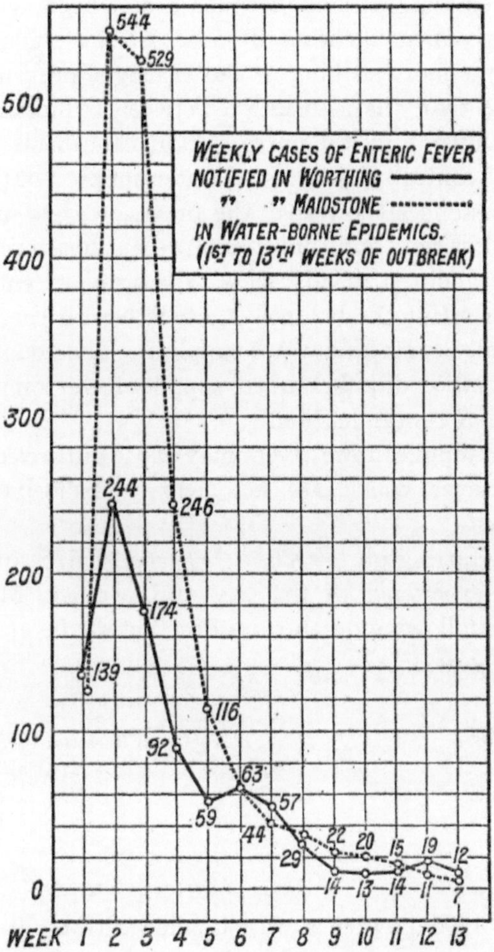

WEEKLY CASES OF ENTERIC FEVER
NOTIFIED IN WORTHING
" " MAIDSTONE
IN WATER-BORNE EPIDEMICS.
(1ST TO 13TH WEEKS OF OUTBREAK)
500
400
300
200
100
0
WEEK 1 2 3 4 5 6 7 8 9 10 11 12 13
544
529
244
246
174
139
116
92
63
59
57
44
29
22
20
15
19
12
14
13
14
11
7


FIG. 6

had been recently fouled; Worthing's supply was from deep wells, in one of which a new heading was being driven at the time of onset of the epidemic. Nothing is more striking in the history of preventive medicine than the association between reduction of enteric fever and the introduction of central and officially controlled sources of water supply: but the above instances show that the provision thus made may, unless rigid and continuous precautionary measures are adopted, vastly widen the scope of enteric infection. But the balance is altogether on the side of centrally controlled water supplies. The adoption of chlorination of public water supplies has minimised this risk of contamination.

Water supplies from rivers may cause outbreaks of enteric fever which are not acutely explosive in character.

Thus Harrington (*Practical Hygiene*, p. 375) quoting the experience of the city of Lawrence, Mass. gives the following death rates from enteric fever in a series of years.

| | *Death rates per 10,000* |
|---|---|
| 1889–1892 | between 13.4 and 10.5 |
| 1893 | 8.0 |
| 1894 | 4.7 |
| 1895 | 3.1 |
| 1896 | 1.9 |
| 1897 | 1.6 |

Prior to 1893 Lawrence was supplied with unfiltered water from the River Merrimac below the point where it received the sewage of large towns. In 1893 a system of water filtration was adopted.

The experience of London is most instructive as regards water-borne disease. In relation to the incidence of cholera the facts are given on page 143 of *Evolution of Preventive Medicine.* But for many years London's water supply from the rivers Thames and Lea has been filtered slowly through sand and gravel beds; and on this precaution and on the purifying effect of large reservoirs by allowing sedimentation of foreign matter, the protection of some millions of people has safely depended. In recent years the further precaution of chlorination of the water has been taken on a considerable scale, as by this means not only is additional protection given, but strain on the working capacity of storage reservoirs is avoided.

This is a convenient point for summarising the history of methods of water purification.

### METHODS OF WATER PURIFICATION

In London in 1608 Sir Hugh Myddleton began the construction of the New River, which brought water to some parts of London by an immense canal from a part of Hertfordshire relatively free from contamination. To him London is immensely indebted. His action carried into practice the best method of water supply,—the supply of water from an uncontaminated source, the area of which can be protected and supervised; and this best method has been adopted by large towns in many countries. Thus in Britain, Liverpool and Birmingham bring their water from lakes in Wales, Manchester from lakes in Westmoreland and Glasgow from Loch Katrine. Many towns are so circumstanced, however, that they must accept water from suspected or recognisably contaminated sources.

Filtration of a portion of the Metropolitan water supply derived from the River Thames was begun in 1829, and it was gradually extended after the cholera epidemic in 1839. In 1855 filtration was made compulsory for all river water distributed to London.

It has been found that for fairly clean waters slow filtration through sand suffices. For muddy water previous sedimentation is needed, or the use of mechanical filters. Lawrence, Mass. had the first American slow sand filter scientifically designed in 1890, Mills, Sedgwick and Hazen being responsible for its installation. Three years earlier the Lawrence Experimental Station had been established, with W. T. Sedgwick as its consulting biologist. He and his colleagues made valuable contributions to the science of water filtration and sewage purification. In America the use of mechanical filters rapidly extended, the filtration being aided by adding a chemical coagulant. Whipple states that in towns with a population over 2500, 30,000 people were being supplied in 1880 with filtered water; in 1920 the population thus supplied exceeded 20 millions.

Chlorination of water was tried in England as early

as 1880. Woodhead first recommended its use in Maidstone in 1897, for disinfecting the water mains after an outbreak of enteric fever. In 1908 it began to be used for purification of water supplies on a large scale. In Jersey City 40 million gallons were thus treated daily about that time: and its use has spread in many countries. In the Great War all medical officers were instructed that 23 grains of chloride of lime would sterilize 100 gallons of clean water in half an hour, suspended matter, if any, being removed previously by the addition of 3 grains of alum to each gallon of water (*Medical History of the War*, vol. 1). Prior to this, filtration of water through earthenware candles had been depended on for field service, and found unsatisfactory, owing to difficulties of transport, slowness of filtration and breakages.

As evidence of the value of chlorine in increasing the safety of water supplies Winslow (*Evolution of Modern Public Health*, p. 38) gives the following figures. A group of 35 large American cities *all* had an enteric fever death rate of over 15 per 100,000 in 1896–1908, while a group of 15 cities at the same period had an enteric death rate of 30 or over. In 1917–1919 only two of the above had an enteric fever death rate over 15, and only 1 a rate over 30 per 100,000.

## VEHICLES OF ENTERIC FEVER OTHER THAN WATER

In the past many outbreaks of enteric fever have been caused by milk to which contaminated water had been added. The first was recognised in 1858 and is mentioned on page 139 of *Evolution of Preventive Medicine*. In 1870 Ballard traced an outbreak of enteric fever in Islington, London, to a particular milk service. Among the 140 families supplied from this dairy 70 attacks and 30 deaths occurred, the disease picking out the milk consumers. Dirty water subject to contamination had been used for dairy purposes.

In 1873 N. Ratcliffe and W. H. Power traced a large outbreak of enteric fever to the milk from a dairy in the west of London, and it was shown that the water in the dairy had excremental contamination. Other outbreaks have been traced to contaminated ice and to ice creams.

### SHELL FISH AND ENTERIC FEVER

In March, 1894, I first drew official notice to oysters as a frequent source of enteric fever in Brighton, and in December, 1894, an outbreak having a similar origin at Wesleyan College, Connecticut was investigated by Conn. Cameron had some years previously suggested this source of enteric fever in Dublin. Sir W. Broadbent drew attention to similar cases in January, 1895, in London. In Brighton at least 30 per cent of the total cases were traced by me to sewage contaminated oysters or mussels. The evidence on which this ascription was based was circumstantial. The shell fish had been consumed within the known period of incubation; shell-fish were proved to be derived from layings in which they were exposed to contamination from sewage; in the affected family only those taking the shell fish were affected, though in some instances those who partook escaped illness, or had only an attack of gastro-enteritis (Gaertner poisoning) occurring much sooner after ingestion of the oysters or mussels than enteric fever having the same origin.

These early observations were later confirmed by outbreaks of enteric fever on a considerable scale where a group of diners had simultaneously eaten contaminated oysters. Thus on November 10, 1902, after Mayoral Banquets at Winchester and Southampton at which there were 267 guests, Bulstrode found that 28 cases of enteric fever and 118 of gastro-enteritis had occurred. The oysters had been grown in uncontaminated layings, but had just before their use been laid down in polluted sea water in the neighborhood of Emsworth. Cockles have similarly been shown by Darra Mair to be largely responsible for the excess of enteric fever occurring in Belfast. A report by Dr. Lumsden and others, on behalf of the United States Public Health Service, describes an extensive prevalence of enteric fever (1924–1925) in a number of American cities, attributable to similarly contaminated oysters.

The history of enteric fever in England shows that, following the general installation of protected water supplies, a rapid decline of the disease occurred. Then the rate of decline slackened up to and including

1899, when a second period of more rapid decline of the disease began and has continued. Between 1894 and 1899 there was much scepticism as to oysters or other shell-fish causing enteric fever; and it was only after simultaneous human experimentation on the scale of public banquets had proved the connection, that diffidence in eating shell-fish and reform in the growing of them became effective. Much of this more rapid decline in the incidence of enteric fever since 1900 has doubtless been caused by the reduction of risk in eating shell-fish. But another factor has been in operation to which attention must be drawn.

### THE "CARRIER" PROBLEM

As indicated on page 49 the contest between an invading microbe and the imperfectly resistant recipient is not necessarily associated with destruction of the invaders as well as the establishment of immunity in the recovered patient. The microbe may continue to survive in its host, and this survival may be a source of danger to the non-immune section of the community. Not only so, but a person may harbour the microbes of diphtheria or cerebrospinal fever, for instance, without falling ill from either of these diseases, and without having suffered from a prior recognisable attack. Evidently these facts complicate the problem of abolition of infectious diseases; though their recognition, as will shortly be seen, has led to the institution of precautionary measures which previously would have been neglected to the damage of the community.

The importance of the "carrier" was first recognised in diphtheria; though earlier than this, in 1881, Pasteur and Sternberg had showed the presence of virulent microörganisms in healthy mouths, subsequently shown to be pneumococci. Roux and Yersin in 1889 drew attention to the persistence of Klebs-Löffler bacilli for considerable periods in the throats of diphtheria convalescents. In 1894 Park and Beebe found diphtheria bacilli in the throats of well persons; and this observation has often been repeated. Epidemiological observations do not give a high place to these carrier case bacilli in provoking local outbreaks of diphtheria, though they cannot be ignored. After an epidemic of diphtheria in a school, many carriers may be discovered among children who have escaped attack; these carriers are often found when Schick tested to have developed immunity.

During the Great War outbreaks of cerebrospinal fever occurred in barracks where there was overcrowding, and attempts were made to segregate well persons who were harbouring meningococci, and even to disinfect the mucous membranes of the nose and throat. The futility of the procedure was indicated when it was found that in sample groups in which no cases of cerebrospinal fever had occurred there were meningococcus carriers in considerable proportions, as well as in invaded groups. The one measure which was most successful in keeping down the proportion of carriers and preventing outbreaks of cerebrospinal fever was adequate spacing out in dormitories.

In dysentery, poliomyelitis and encephalitis lethargica the problem of the carrier also arises.

H. S. Hartley in 1900 drew attention to the urinary carrier of typhoid bacilli. Koch in 1902 emphasised the importance of the typhoid carrier as an epidemiological factor, and stressed the importance of disinfection of excreta and urine of patients, as also of inquiring as to the occurrence of ambulant and abortive cases of enteric fever, especially in children. A South German campaign organised by Koch was undertaken on these lines, systematic exmination of urine and foeces being undertaken. Before this it had been demonstrated that typhoid bacilli may persist even for years in the gall bladder or be found in a chronic periosteal abscess. In 1904 Drigalski showed that typhoid bacilli may be present in the foeces of persons who have apparently never had enteric fever.

Such carriers are particularly dangerous if they are concerned in the handling of food for others. Two instances of this are well known. Kayser describes the case of a Strasburg's baker's wife whose apprentice died from enteric fever in May, 1904, and each apprentice in succession had an attack of this disease. The baker's wife was found to be a carrier: she had gone through an attack of enteric fever ten years earlier.

Drs. Davies and Walker Hall described an outbreak of enteric fever at an Inebriate Reformatory in Bristol, in which there were 240 inmates and 24 resident staff. There had been no enteric fever in the institution since it was opened; but in September 1899 a kitchen helper fell ill with this disease, and in November three more cases were recognised. In the following May one case, in June none, in July six, in August nine, in September one, in October two and in November four cases occurred. Milk was suspected, but all milk drunk had been boiled. One inmate a helper aged 50, however, handled the milk after it had been sterilised and gave it out to the patients. She was found to be a carrier and on further inquiries it was discovered that she had apparently been responsible for previous outbreaks of enteric fever in two other institutions.

On account of this risk systematic examination of workers in restaurants is enforced as a routine in some American cities. If the examination of these workers is adequate (including several bacteriological examinations of excreta) it affords some protection: if not it may give a false sense of security. The importance of such examinations is especially great for men or women who have had an acute illness which may have been enteric fever or gastro-enteritis.

It may be well to mention in concluding this incomplete sketch of an important subject that "carriers" of infection, i.e., carriers at other times than during an attack of the disease in question, occur in three connections: (*a*) Primary or precocious carriers, who excrete the bacillus during the incubation period of disease; (*b*) the infectious contact, e.g., a nurse or attendant on the sick, who never suffers from an attack of the disease; and (*c*) the chronic carrier, with whom the preceding paragraphs are chiefly concerned.

So far as the last named is concerned, little or no success has been secured in ridding the gall bladder from typhoid bacilli by medicinal means or operations; and apart from operation on tonsils and adenoids the chronic carrier of diphtheria bacilli has resisted treatment successfully.

### DEFECTIVE SANITARY ARRANGEMENTS

Little stress has been laid in preceding paragraphs on insanitation as directly provocative of enteric fever. It is evident, however, that if human excremental matter is kept in pails or privies near houses there may be spillings of their contents, and flies may carry infection to milk or other foods. In towns there has been a steady reduction of enteric fever in proportion as a water-carriage system of disposal of excreta has been adopted, and pails and privies have been abandoned. The usually coincident improvement in water supply has been even more concerned; but that even with a good water supply imperfect domestic sanitation may mean excessive incidence of typhoid fever has been repeatedly demonstrated.

In the American Army Camps in 1898 and still more in the Boer War 1899–1900 great importance was attached to flies as carrying the infection of enteric fever and of dysentery to food. In the circumstances of these campaigns there is no doubt that such convection of infection occurred; but I am inclined to agree with the late Sir George Turner (*British Medical Journal*, February 15, 1902) in deprecating the tendency to rest content with wind and flies as responsible for spreading enteric fever. Many cases thus attributed were almost certainly caused by contaminated water; and in other instances direct infection from comrade to comrade or from patient to attendant occurred. Whenever the nursing of enteric fever has been carried out with inadequate or unskilled help, there has been spread of this disease by direct contact.

# CHAPTER XII

## The Prevention of Undulant (Malta or Mediterranean) Fever

Although this disease is almost unknown in Britain, and has been regarded as almost unknown elsewhere except where goats are kept (see page 110) its prevention forms an especially instructive chapter in the history of preventive medicine. As events actually developed the discovery of its causal microbe formed an indispensable link in ascertaining its causation, and it is probable that the success of the epidemiological investigation which resulted in the discovery of milk as probably the sole vector of infection would have been long retarded but for the serological tests which the discovery of the *Micrococcus melitensis* made practicable. In the *Transactions of the Epidemiological Society of London*, 1889–1890 Malta fever was described as a "dirt fever" due to poisonous emanations from Malta's tideless and sewage-contaminated harbour. At this time Bruce's discovery of the *Mic. melit.* was already known.

Malta fever is a severe disease; two per cent of the British troops and sailors attacked by it died. It involved hospital treatment on an average for 120 days, and sometimes had sequelæ lasting two or even more years. During the illness itself the patient had long continued fever and severe joint pains, and was reduced to a state of great emaciation and weakness from which recovery was slow.

In a statement published in 1908 (*The Extinction of Malta Fever* (Research Defence Society, 1908)) Sir David Bruce stated that the soldiers in Malta numbered about 700 and that undulant fever was responsible on an average for 312 admissions to hospital annually and about the same number of sailors, implying a total of 75,000 days of illness per annum. For many years this disease had been made the subject of clinical and epidemiological study. It was more common among officers and women than among non-commissioned officers and men, and it had no apparent relation to sanitary conditions. It also occurred very considerably not only in Malta but also in other parts of the Mediterranean and elsewhere. It was shown that water was not the source of infection.

In 1887 Bruce found the *Mic. melitensis* in the blood of patients; and this organism after isolation from the spleen-pulp of several fatal human cases was found to fulfil the postulates of Koch. Bruce proved its etiological importance by experimentation on monkeys; which after inoculation developed the symptoms of undulant fever. Somewhat later specific agglutinins were found in infected animals and in patients; and the application of the tests thereby made available facilitated the subsequent investigations which proved the channel of infection of the disease. It was also found that the *Mic. melitensis* does not increase outside the body, and that in a few hours it is destroyed by sunlight, though it is more persistent of vitality in the shade. Dust was eliminated as a source of infection by the examination with negative results of large quantities of the air in fever wards and in drains and sewers. The deposit from such air tested on animals always failed to produce the disease. Epidemiological work had already shown that it did not spread from the patient to those in attendance on him and that water supply was not concerned. Mosquitoes were also eliminated as a source of infection.

In 1905 W. H. Horrocks found the *Mic. melitensis* in the milk of apparently healthy goats; and further investigations showed that blood serum derived from goats in the island usually gave positive agglutination results when tested against the *Mic. melitensis.* Horrocks later showed that at Gibraltar Malta fever disappeared when, owing to the expense of importation, Maltese goats ceased to be imported, and Spanish goats were substituted.

The previous experimental results clearly indicated that the parasite causing this disease depended on some warm-blooded animal for its continued existence. Feeding experiments showed that the disease could be communicated to monkeys and kids by contaminating various foods with cultures of *Mic. melitensis;* and goats' milk as a staple food in Malta came under suspicion. In Malta there was one goat to every 10 of the population. Then inoculation experiments were made. Several goats when inoculated with *Mic. melitensis* showed no signs of ill health, though a week or two later their blood contained this organism; and their blood serum gave the same positive agglutination test as did a patient suffering or recovered from undulant fever. Further investigations of some thousands of the goats in the island showed that half of them responded to the agglutination test, and that ten per cent were secreting *Mic. melitensis* in their milk. This organism was also found in the blood and in urine excreted by these goats.

On the 19th of August 1905 an unintentional human experiment clinched the conclusion that goats' milk conveyed the infection of Malta fever. Some 61 milch goats and 4 bill goats were exported from Malta to America on *S.S. Joshua Nicholson*. They appeared to be healthy and were good milkers. The milk of these goats was drunk freely by the crew of 23 men. About 13 of these there is no evidence; but of the remaining ten 9 had febrile attacks, 5 showing definite evidence of undulant fever. The goats were killed on arriving in America, and 32 of them were found to be infected.

Even without this dramatic confirmation, the aggregate previous investigations, checked as they were by experimental blood tests, proved that goats' milk was a means of transmitting undulant fever; and the only remaining doubt was as to whether its mode of spread could be narrowed down to this single path, or whether it might also be communicated otherwise.

Immediate steps were taken to stop the supply of goats' milk to the troops and naval forces in the Mediterranean, or to have it always boiled. In Malta preventive measures began in June, 1906, with results which may be thus summarized.

*Malta fever in forces in Malta*

| | *Incidence per 1000* |
|---|---|
| In the 6 years 1899–1905 | 27.6* |
| In the 1st 6 months of 1906 | 31.0 |
| In the 2nd 6 months of 1906 | 11.0 |

* Average.

After that it disappeared from Malta with dramatic suddenness. The goats still harboured the causal agent of the disease, but the disease was eliminated, when once the channel of its transmission was blocked.

Recent investigations have shown that disease due to the *Mic. melitensis* or to an organism almost indistinguishable from it is somewhat widely spread in the western states of America. Outbreaks have occurred where goats are kept; and evidence is accumulating that the bacillus producing abortion in cattle is intimately connected with similar outbreaks, which may occur apart from infection by goats' milk. Human cases of undulant fever are also reported in the States, in which infection appears to have been derived from cows' milk and in some instances from contact with dejecta or other material from infected cattle or hogs.

# CHAPTER XIII

## THE PREVENTION OF LOUSE-BORNE DISEASES

In temperate climates the three chief diseases in this group are relapsing fever, typhus fever and trench fever.

*Relapsing fever* has become extinct in Britain, except for a rare imported case. In the earlier part of the 19th century it was not uncommon, though confused with other forms of fever. It was nearly always associated with circumstances of privation and crowding: hence its name of "famine fever." The spirillum of relapsing fever was discovered by Obermeier in 1873, and in 1878 Vandyke Carter found this spirillum in the blood of relapsing fever patients in India. He was able to reproduce the disease by inoculating small monkeys. In Russia the disease had been common, and in that country bugs have been credited with spreading it. It is now known that it is spread by the louse, not by its bite, but by escape of the parasite from the body of the crushed louse, and its entry into man through excoriations of the skin. The disease, as its name indicates, is characterised by return of the fever after an interval. During this interval spirochetes are absent from the blood. The disease is at once arrested by the administration of salvarsan or neo-salvarsan. In this respect it resembles syphilis, another spirochetal disease (page 171).

*Typhus fever* has already been considered with some fullness in Chapter XV and XVI of *Evolution of Preventive Medicine* and we need only consider here its more modern history. In the official statistics for England and Wales it was only tabulated separately from typhoid fever from 1869 onwards.

| *England and Wales.* | *Number of deaths from typhus fever* |
|---|---|
| 1st period—15 years (1869–1887) | 23,702 |
| 2nd period—15 years (1884–1898) | 2,249 |
| 3rd period—15 years (1889–1913) | 390 |
| 4th period—15 years (1914–1924) | 32 |

The story of the reduction of typhus fever must be read in the light of two outstanding facts. This reduction, amounting almost to disappearance in Britain occurred: (1) before it was known that typhus is spread and probably is spread only by the louse; and (2) before we had any knowledge of the bacteriology of the disease. With this in mind we may next state our knowledge on these two points. Nicolle and co-workers in 1909 first reported the transmission of typhus by the bite of the *Pediculus vestimenti* (body louse) to monkeys and from monkey to monkey. Their work was suggested by the previous successful work of Sergent with relapsing fever. They showed that the fœces of lice infected with typhus were infective. The relative share of these and of inoculation by bite in man is perhaps still uncertain.

In New York and in other parts of the United States there has appeared a milder form of typhus fever

(Brill's disease). The symptoms of the two appear to be identical, and Brill's disease follows the same though a milder course than ordinary typhus. In both, the so-called Weil-Felix reaction is given.

This western disease does not appear to occur in epidemics and it appears not to spread from man to man. It is doubtful if body lice are its sole vectors. Brill has reported a considerable number of cases in New York. If this account is correct, a new sanitary problem is raised, with suggested analogies in typhoid and paratyphoid, in small pox and alastrim. The monkey has been shown to be susceptible to this variety as well as to the ordinary typhus, and in 1910 Ricketts and Wilder while confirming this observation for the Mexican typhus have shown the possibility of its transmission by the louse. They have also described the presence in the blood of bacillus-like organisms now known as *Rickettsia Prowazek.* It is possible that the Mexican typhus is a third variety differing from Brill's disease. The Public Health Reports of the United States Public Health Service for December 24, 1926, contain an important contribution by Dr. K. F. Maxcy, on "Endemic Typhus (Brill's Disease) in the South Eastern United States" in which doubt is thrown on the man-to-man transference by lice of this possibly third disease, and it is suggested that there may be a reservoir of this disease in rodents, from which the disease is occasionally transmitted to man.

So far as the typhus of temperate climates is concerned it is fairly certain that the virus is conveyed from man to man only by the agency of the louse, in which the unknown parasite of typhus passes through a cycle of about five days before the disease can be further transmitted.

This being so, the history of typhus must be read in the light of this biological fact. Slums have been cleared on an extensive scale in our cities, bringing in fresh air and light. Personal cleanliness has vastly improved as has also the whitewashing of bedrooms and diminution of overcrowding. Thorne stated that between 1856 and 1887 over 14 millions sterling were devoted in London to operations by the Metropolitan Board of Works tending "almost exclusively to the destruction of unwholesome house property." In the same way the gradual removal of "back-to-back" houses which were without through ventilation has helped, as has also the prohibition of sleeping in cellar dwellings. Nevertheless the two main factors which have led to the rapid disappearance of typhus must have been (1) the diminution of lousiness, and (2) the prevention of the passage of lice from typhus patients to others.

The second of these conditions implies that "fever" hospitals have been extremely important in bringing about the disappearance of typhus.

The place and share of importance of the first is illustrated by the history of typhus in the Great War. Napoleonic troops returning from Russia, and most armies in earlier centuries have been decimated by "camp fever." Similarly it decimated large masses of population on and behind the Eastern front in the Great War. It began in Servia in 1915 and by April of that year the deaths in a day amounted up to 9000. Why were the Western troops of the allies free from typhus? This immunity has been ascribed to the cleansing of men and their clothing which was carried out on a gigantic scale. But in the first year of the war, owing to the sudden aggregation of millions of men in improvised huts and camps, often without means of ablution or change of shirts, both scabies and pediculosis prevailed to a painful extent in large masses of troops: and the organisation for "de-lousing" on a fairly adequate scale was a task of months and even of years. The men got trench fever—also a louse borne disease—right to the end of the war. But they escaped typhus; and one must infer that,—in part owing to lack of communication across the lines with Russian troops, in part owing to general stoppage of communication with typhus-infested countries,—typhus was never introduced in a sufficient number of cases to form foci of infection.

This experience, indeed, furnishes an excellent text for a homily as to the multiplicity of factors required to cause an epidemic of an acutely infectious disease. Failure to diagnose early cases, failure to isolate every known case, failure to search out overlooked cases, failure to prevent introduction of infection into a community are all concerned. Of course if every member of the population was free from infestation by lice, this also would suffice to prevent the spread of infection when imported; but this ideal is far from being realised.

*Trench fever* was first identified during the Great War, during which scabies and trench fever with its sequelæ were responsible for more absence from military duty than any other infection on the Western Front. The amount of wastage of man-power produced by trench fever has been estimated at from one-fifth to one-third of the total illness of the British Armies in France. The history of trench fever somewhat resembles that of undulant fever, with the important distinction that the infecting parasite,—believed by some to be a filter-passing organism—has not yet been discovered. It is probably an ancient disease, not confined to military life, and may be responsible for many of the cases of "febricula," which were common in the early days when enteric and typhus fever were confused. It is characterised by recurrent fever, each attack lasting some 5 or 6 days. In some cases febrile relapses occur after months of quiescence.

Bryan and his associates in their investigation of trench fever found that the bite of an infected louse did not suffice to transmit this disease, but that it could be communicated when the excreta of infected lice were rubbed into the scarified skin; also that the excreta only became infective 7 days or more after having fed on a patient. This suggests a developmental cycle, part of which is passed in the louse; and this may be so also for typhus. The lice, they found, remained infective for at least 23 days; and an infected louse is now stated to excrete active virus for the remainder of its life.

McKnee and his fellow-workers showed in 1916 that volunteers could be inoculated successfully with trench fever by means of blood of fever patients. The infectious blood ceased to infect after filtration through a Berkefeld filter. In 1917 Pappenheimer and Mueller of New York transmitted the disease to one of three volunteers by allowing lice to feed on trench fever patients and then on these volunteers. A patient's blood may remain infective as late as the 300th day after attack by the disease. The experiments, some of the results of which are imperfectly summarised above, were made on volunteers for the purpose; and these were kept under conditions precluding other sources of trench fever. Trench fever was not at once recognised as a separate entity during the Great War, and among the British soldiers it was not made notifiable until 1918. Exact statistics are therefore not attainable; but there appears to be no doubt that although it has seldom proved fatal, some cases have become chronic with disordered heart action, and that during the war it was a major cause of disability as already indicated. And it would have been absent, had it been possible to keep the soldiers clean, while its amount would have been relatively small had infestation with body-lice been less common than was the case.

Relapsing fever, typhus fever, and now trench fever are thus diseases of social misery, because under such conditions infection becomes more common and occurs in larger dosage, because in such circumstances neither is the person washed nor his clothing washed and changed, and because the closeness of individual contact, with the continuously higher temperature of such contact conduces to the multiplication of vermin. But, as in the case of typhus the distribution of lice-borne diseases does not correspond exactly with that of lice. Pediculosis is prevalent among school-children, notwithstanding the steady beneficent work of school hygienists which is reducing it; and it has been shown that pediculus capitis can convey trench fever. Probably this is true also for typhus fever. Among the British soldiers, who suffered from pediculus corporis, typhus as we have seen, was unknown, in striking contrast to the experience of Russian, Polish and Serbian armies, and of German soldiers when they come into contact with these. Evidently, therefore, the introduction of infection is necessary, and carelessness in respect of isolation of patients, of surveillance of contacts, or failure to recognise the disease, is implied when typhus fever spreads.

Trench fever and typhus alike may be taken to illustrate the lesson that even when the source of infection cannot be directly attacked, the links connecting case with case can be broken, with the result that in the end the disease ceases to spread. This indeed is the general rôle of applied preventive medicine. Whether we are concerned with typhus or enteric fever, with measles or whooping cough, with trench fever or malaria, the work of the hygienist consists in blocking the routes of infection, in rendering them impassable, and thereby, so to speak, destroying the disease by inanition. Exceptions where other lines of action are practicable are furnished in small-pox, enteric fever, diphtheria and possibly yellow fever, in which susceptible persons can be rendered insusceptible by vaccinal processes; but the triumphs of preventive medicine on these lines are relatively few, though most important. So far as enteric fever in civilian urban life in any country is concerned, we should think of anti-typhoid vaccination as a *pis aller*, not to be recommended for the general population, but only to nurses and others who are exposed to immediate and repeated possibilities of infection. (See also page 78).

# CHAPTER XIV

## Hookworm Disease (Ankylostomiasis)

So far our account of individual preventible diseases has been concerned with diseases which are either (*a*) transmissible from man to man by ingestion or inhalation, (enteric fever and small pox) or (*b*) transmissible from animals to man by inoculation through abrasions or by a bite (anthrax and rabies) or (*c*) in which inoculation is effected by body lice, (typhus, trench fever and relapsing fever).

In this chapter hookworm disease is considered. The infecting agent of this disease in its embryonic stage bores its way through the human skin; and this disease illustrates, perhaps better than any other disease the close relationship between defective sanitation and disease. It is caused by a parasite whose life-history is completely known, and which can be conquered both on preventive and curative lines. And yet with the possible exceptions of malaria, syphilis, tuberculosis and cancer it is, when internationally considered, one of the most serious diseases of mankind; not so much as a cause of death as by producing serious physical and mental disablement. Persons infested with the worms, the attacks of which cause the symptoms of this disease, suffer from anæmia, gastro-intestinal disturbance, boils, nettle-rash, and toxæmia. The abdomen becomes distended, and physiological development is delayed and diminished. A boy of sixteen may have the appearance and development of one of ten. The victims of this disease are apathetic and feeble both in body and mind. The symptoms are somewhat in proportion to the number of hookworms harboured. Thus in observations in Alabama 100 hookworms or more produced definite mental and physical retardation in children aged 6 to 18. If there were fewer than 25 hookworms no measurable symptoms appeared. The worm producing these symptoms is small and belongs to one of two species, *Ankylostoma duodenalis*, the old world type, or *Necator Americanus*, the new world type. The latter is said to be the more active and destructive, though both worms produce a general profound anæmia and resultant lack of nutrition for physical and mental growth. The adult female worm is about ½ inch in length, the male about ⅓ inch. They attach themselves to the mucous membrane of the intestine, especially of the jejune, it may be in thousands, and greedily absorb blood from the small wounds which they make in the mucous membrane. A worm does not remain fixed to one site, and with each bite not only is there further bleeding but additional points are left for toxic and bacterial absorption. The adult females produce an enormous number of eggs over long periods, and in a case of serious infestation four million eggs may be evacuated daily in the host's fœces. A mature female may discharge 5000 eggs in a day.

The eggs are only visible under the microscope. Their further development requires access to the open air, moisture and a warm temperature. When discharged on to a suitable soil larvae from $\frac{1}{125}$ to $\frac{1}{100}$ inch in length develop in two days. They double their length in a week. The further development of these larvae, which are motile, depends on their gaining access to their human host, either through the skin, or more exceptionally by the mouth in drinking water, or solid food, or from contaminated fingers.

Looss in Cairo in 1895 accidentally discovered that the skin was the channel of infection. He spilled a drop of water containing many encysted larvae on his hand, and found that they disappeared, leaving their delicate sheaths behind them. Some 71 days later he developed definite uncinariasis (hookworm infestation). In a volunteer the same sequence was observed, evidence of intestinal infestation being obtained in 74 days. The parasites usually pierce though a hair follicle, commonly between the toes, producing symptoms known as "ground itch."

The larvae travelling in the blood to the right side of the heart are too large to pass through the capillaries of the lung. They penetrate the alveoli of the lung, and after wandering up the trachea to the throat are swallowed and finally lodge in the intestine, where they begin the next stage in their maleficent life-cycle.

Hookworm disease only prevails in certain circumstances. The hookworms flourish in the sandy soil of the Southern States. In Tennessee they are harmless. Shade, moisture, and a warm temperature—57° to 99°F.—are needed to favor their extra-corporeal development. The larvae do not hatch out much below 50°F. These facts explain the almost total freedom from the disease in Western Europe, with occasional exceptions in mines and in the boring of tunnels, in which the temperature is relatively high.

In 1883 an outbreak of so-called "miners' anæmia" occurred among the laborers engaged in the St. Gothard's tunnel, Switzerland, and similar outbreaks of hookworm disease have occurred in mines of England, Germany, and South Africa. An outbreak in a Cornish mine at Dolcoath was described by Boycott and J. S. Haldane (*Journal of Hygiene*, vol. iii, 1903). There was no privy accommodation underground. Ova of hookworms were found in fœcal deposits, which must have been trodden on. It is likely that the infection had been introduced by miners who had returned from similar work in subtropical countries.

The natural history of this disease unmistakably teaches that the most effective means for preventing it consists in elementary sanitation. The disease is acquired chiefly by the class of persons who, in hot climates, go about with bare feet, and thus come into contact with the embryoes of the hookworm. A conceivable alternative method of prevention would be that neither man, woman nor child should walk except in shoes; but this obviously is impracticable to enforce, and if it were attempted the compulsory wearing of shoes would be an uneconomic method of safeguarding against infection.

Dr. J. A. Farrell (*American Journal of Public Health*, February, 1920) has revealed a state of matters which implies the continuance on a large scale of this disease. He states that of some 96,000 houses examined in 236 rural areas in the Southern part of the United States only 9.8 per cent had adequate latrine accommodation, and 5.3 per cent had none. Colonel Stiles of the American Public Health Service, who has been a pioneer in anti-hookworm work, has always emphasised the provision and use of satisfactory privies with pits as the prime need in this connection. Stiles has estimated that two million persons are infested with hookworms along the American littoral and the Gulf States, between the Potomac and the Mississippi. The valuable anti-hookworm work organised by the Rockefeller Sanitary Commission (subsequently the International Health Board)—the beneficent activities of which have extended to many countries,—appears to have been activated in the first instance by Stiles' investigations. The essential first principle in the prevention of hookworm disease is the provision for every family of a cheap fool-proof latrine. It should preferably be movable, the pit being adequately covered when the wooden framework of the privy is moved.

Other measures which are of value are suggested by our knowledge of the hookworm. Doubtful drinking water should be boiled, and the hands should be washed before preparing or eating food.

Treatment plays an important part in the prevention of this disease. The provision of gratuitous treatment forms an important public health measure. Such treatment not only hastens the cure of the patient; it also gives an opportunity to educate patients as to the disease, as to latrine provision, and as to personal cleanliness.

Treatment,—for which thymol, oil of chenopodium, and carbon tetrachloride have been found to be efficient,—even when it stops short of complete elimination of the worms, greatly improves the health of the infested person, making him capable of economic work. It also greatly reduces the risk of infection to others.

This disease, in tropical and sub-tropical climates, may be said to be an index of sanitary civilisation. The preventive work already done in many countries has had a most salutory effect; but relapses occur, due to economic difficulties and to the people themselves, and this must be expected. That ere long, however, this devitalising disease will be controlled to a rapidly increasing extent cannot be doubted.

## CHAPTER XV

### The Prevention of Plague

The earlier history of plague and of the pre-scientific attempts at its control has been sketched in Chapter X of *Evolution of Preventive Medicine.* The story of the unfolding of our knowledge of its natural history and of the rational preventive measures now based on this knowledge is a romance in preventive medicine, which is briefly outlined in this chapter. Although plague continues to be one of the most devastating of the world's diseases, our knowledge of its causation and methods of spread is now so complete as to render its continued prevalence no longer inevitable.

There is no evidence of the autocthonous origin of plague in Europe. It has always been imported from the East, coming in pandemics at intervals the rationale of which is mysterious. The Black Death of the fourteenth century was the greatest plague experienced by Christendom: it has been stated that in Europe with a population of some 25 millions, one-fourth disappeared during this pandemic.

A pandemic prevailed in the seventeenth century in Europe, Asia and Africa, and then it gradually receded for a century and a half. In 1845 it had disappeared from Egypt, although that country for many years had been an epidemic center.

The Bills of Mortality of London for three epidemic years during the seventeenth century may be quoted:

*London*

| Year | Total deaths from all causes | Deaths from plague |
|---|---|---|
| 1625 | 54,265 | 35,417 |
| 1636 | 23,359 | 10,400 |
| 1665 | 97,306 | 68,596 |

The most recent pandemic appears to have started in China, where it has prevailed as an endemic in Yannan since 1870. Since 1894 plague has spread throughout the world, though its chief incidence has been in India, China, the Philippines and Mauritius.

In most areas the spread of plague has been slow and insidious; and it has seldom been possible to state how it was introduced into a given country. In an earlier pandemic, the Great Plague of London, 1665, was the culmination of smaller epidemics during some 70 years.

In India the deaths registered from plague in the years 1896 to 1909 inclusive numbered 6,308,650. In 1896 only 2,288 deaths were returned as caused by plague: in 1903 the number had increased to 1,112,376, in 1907 to 1,318,880, the number declining to 150,756 in 1908.

Since the years immediately following the Great Plague England has been free from plague, except for occasional imported cases. The reason for this will be better understood when the recent additions to our knowledge of the causation of plague have been stated.

In 1894 the *Bacillus pestis* was discovered by Kitasato and Yersin in the blood and tissues of plague patients; and inasmuch as (1) the microörganism is always found in the lesions of the patient, before and after his death; (2) this microörganism can be isolated from the patient and cultured; (3) plague can be transmitted to guinea pigs or rats by inoculation of material from these cultures; and lastly (4) the same microörganism is always found subsequently in these animals, the specific causal relation of this micro-organism to plague is established.

Prior to the work of the Indian Plague Commission, whose reports were published in the *Journal of Hygiene* (1906–1910), it had become clear that plague rarely spread from man to man, except in the rare pneumonic form of the disease; also that plague was not readily contracted by eating or drinking infected material; and that the occurrence of plague in man was generally, and probably always, preceded by an outbreak of the disease among rats, more rarely among other animals, as the ground squirrel in California, the marmot in Thibet, and the tarbagan—a fur-bearing rodent—in Manchuria.

These epidemiological facts naturally led to the inference that rat plague was connected with plague in man. Rats are great travellers, but their progress is not rapid; and similarly in a given country plague spreads slowly from district to district. It dies down in the winter, and increases in the summer months. The explanation of these phenomena is found in the hypothesis first advocated by Simond in 1897, as the result of his experience in India, that fleas are the intermediary agents for transmitting plague from rats to man.

Ogato in 1897 found plague bacilli in fleas derived from rats dead of bubonic plague; and he gave plague to mice by inoculating them with crushed fleas taken from infected rats.

Simonds' views were advocated by Dr. Ashburton Thompson who advanced facts and considerations in their favor based on his experience of an outbreak of plague in Sydney. Many facts converged in favor of the rat-flea origin of plague in man. Thus the seasonal increase of fleas is followed by an increase of rodent plague; and the Indian Plague Commission in 1908 found that in India fleas cease to multiply at temperatures over 85°F. and plague bacilli disappear from their bodies.

Bacot found that a rat flea which had fed on an infected rat could carry plague bacilli for 47 days, and at the end of this time infect a mouse. He also found that an infected rat can harbour as many as 100 fleas.

The experiments devised by the Indian Plague Commission and carried out by a team of workers cleared up all doubts. It was found that the rat flea (*Xenopsylla cheopis*) is not the same as man's flea (*Pulex irritans*) but that the rat flea will leave an infected rat when it dies, and will then bite a man.

Hence the special danger of handling dead rats before they are cold. Other fleas can convey the infection; but in nature the *X. cheopis* probably is the only flea which transmits plague from rat to rat. A practical inference is that by examining the rats in a port for the extent of their infestation with this flea, there is obtained some measure of the possibilities of plague invasion.

It was also proved that plague bacilli multiply in the flea's stomach. C. J. Martin has shown that the proventriculus of the flea is blocked by a mass of plague bacilli, and that infection of man occurs by regurgitation of infected food from the stomach of the flea during the act of biting.

Experiments made for the Indian Plague Commission showed that rats fed on bodies of rats dead of plague did not become infected, not even when they were fed on the excreta of diseased rats. It was found also that plague rats themselves did not infect the floors of invaded houses; for healthy rats and guinea pigs running about these floors did not acquire plague, so long as fleas were absent. On the other hand failing this condition guinea pigs acquired plague in infected huts, even though the huts had been washed out with perchloride of mercury solution. Clearly neither food nor soil was responsible for the spread of plague.

In hospitals for plague even when there were many fleas, no spread of plague occurred, showing that the human flea is not the agent of infection.

The following experiments are most instructive. Healthy rats having been brought from England, a glass cage was made large enough to hold two rat cages. The enclosing cage was made flea proof by small meshed linen, but this linen was not used for the two cages within. In one of these inner cages a rat inoculated with the plague bacillus was placed along with 20 to 30 rat fleas. When this rat died and was removed, healthy rats were placed in the next inner cage, and these soon died of plague.

The jumping distance of a rat flea is 3 to 5 inches, never over 6 inches. A healthy rat placed in a cage above and beyond the reach of the jump of fleas never took plague; but all rats placed similarly in non-insect-proof cages at a lower level did so. Evidently the flea was the carrier of plague.

Then the plague rats deprived of their fleas were placed in a room with 50 flealess healthy guinea pigs. The floor remained uncleansed, aerial infection if it occurs was possible throughout. All the plague rats died, all the guinea pigs remained well. Thus direct contagion, food and aerial infection were excluded as causing plague.

It was found that houses from which plague patients had been removed were dangerous in proportion to the number of rat fleas. Guinea pigs were allowed to run for 24 hours in such houses, then their fleas were stupified with chloroform, collected and counted. They were more numerous in the plague houses.

The facts, of which an incomplete summary is

given above show that by controlling rats plague can be entirely controlled. There can be no reasonable doubt that pandemic migrations of plague can be controlled as successfully as those of cholera. In neither disease, owing to unrecognised cases and the many possibilities of transport, are attempts at quarantine of human patients and contacts likely to be successful. In cholera what is needed is sanitation and supervision of contacts and suspects within each country; and in plague there is needed persistent attack on rats on a scale which will prevent their invasion of dwelling houses and food stores. In most ports all rats discovered dead are subjected to bacteriological examination, and ships are required to undergo regular deratisation. Various methods to this end are in use; apart from this procedure, the essential points are to diminish the rat population by preventing their access to any food supplies and for this purpose to make dwelling houses and warehouses as far as possible rat-proof.

At this point we may consider in review the three great pandemic diseases which—excluding influenza and possibly typhus—have been the greatest plagues of mankind,—plague, cholera, and small pox. In all three of these the pandemic travels can be overcome by practicable measures. For small pox and cholera this has been done with a large measure of success, and even plague is now seldom serious except in its countries of origin.

In all three the production of artificial immunity

against attack has been practised with some success; in small pox with complete success when intelligently applied. In cholera and in plague, however, one can only regard protective inoculation as of secondary value and importance. Without this it is completely practicable to advance towards extinction of these diseases.

# CHAPTER XVI

## Filariasis and Texas Fever

In our review of the story of modern preventive medicine we come next to the work of Patrick Manson on filariasis and Theobald Smith on Texas Fever, which may be described as pivotal investigations. On them has depended the most dramatic and important advance in preventive medicine made during the last quarter of a century.

These investigations showed that in certain diseases, a portion of the life-history of the contagium is passed in an intermediate insect host (the word "insect" is used in a wider sense than its strict zoological meaning), in which host the contagium passes through some of the changes required to complete its cycle of life. Such changes in the intermediate host have more recently been discovered in the louse in its transmission of trench fever; but the changes occurring in the life-history of diseases of which filariasis and Texas fever may be regarded as the prototype are more extensive than those known to occur in any louse-borne disease.

Before describing these changes, we may briefly refer in contrast to the house fly, as a casual vector of disease. It has been shown to be capable of carrying putrefactive fragments or even specific infective material from fœcal matter to man or to his food.

In 1869 anthrax bacilli were demonstrated on flies fed on specifically infected material. Nuttall in 1897 showed that horse flies can carry plague bacilli for at least 48 hours after being infected. In 1886 cholera spirilla were found in the flies in a cholera hospital. Firth and Horrocks in 1902 demonstrated typhoid bacilli on the legs and bodies of flies. Many other similar results have been recorded. Epidemiologically J. Niven and others have drawn attention to the coincidence in cities between the number of flies and the amount of summer diarrhoea. Whether this is in part merely coincidence with the other changes of temperature etc. in summer or is a real causal relation is open to some doubt.

In armies during war, as in South Africa and in American expeditions, flies are regarded as having played a very important part in spreading typhoid fever among the troops. (On this see also page 105.) But the fly is merely a mechanical vector of septic or infective material, while the flea in plague and the louse in typhus, relapsing fever and trench fever inoculate specific bacterial material.

In the group of diseases next to be considered, filariasis, texas fever, malaria and yellow fever, a cycle of the life history of the vector of infection takes place in a mosquito or tick, which also acts as an inoculator of the infective material. Patrick Manson initiated this new knowledge, which forms the foundation of Tropical Medicine. Born in 1844 and dying in 1922, Manson as a young doctor practised in Amoy, a Chinese port, and there saw cases of elephantiasis with enormously swollen legs. At that time their causation was unknown, although in 1866 Wucherer had found a micro-filaria in the urine of a case of hœmaturia in Brazil and two years later also in patients suffering from hœmatochyluria. Lewis also described what he found in a chyluria patient as follows: "the embryo of a nematoid worm, which may give a clue to one cause of this mysterious malady" (Sanitary Commissioner of India's Report, 1869).

In 1876–1877 Bancroft discovered adult female worms of this micro-filaria in a lymphatic abscess, and Cobbold gave it the name of *Filaria Bancrofti.* Manson while on leave in London in 1874 heard of Lewis's discovery in 1872 of the filaria *Sanguinis hominis* in the blood of inhabitants of some parts of India. Returning to China next year Manson discovered these micro-filariæ in some districts in a proportion of the population varying from 10 to 50 per cent, in other districts in none. He concluded that as the filaria did not grow in the blood it must be an immature form. As the micro-filaria was never found in urine or other natural discharges, Manson inferred that it could not escape from the human body unless helped by a carrying agent which could suck blood through the skin; and in this connection the mosquito at once came under suspicion.

With the help of two native assistants Manson

proceeded to examine the blood of 1000 natives, one assistant working by day and one by night. During the day results were nearly always negative, at night the micro-filaria was commonly found in abstracted blood. Sometimes as many as 200 embryos were found in a single drop of blood. Here was an evident suggestion of adaptation to the nocturnal habits of the mosquito.

The next stage was the discovery of micro-filariæ in blood abstracted by mosquitoes. It was also found that the digestive juices of the mosquito did not kill these filariæ. After many months' further work Manson traced the filarial embryo through the walls of the mosquito's stomach into its abdominal cavity and thence into its thoracic muscles. In this passage the micro-filaria grew enormously and developed an alimentary canal and sex organs. Later the filaria was actually shown in the act of passing through the proboscis of the mosquito, on its way to enter the human system through the mosquito's bite. This journey has been traced by Low, Grassi and Fülleborn. The events thus scantily outlined constituted as will be seen hereafter, an epoch making discovery, of untold value to the human race.

It is possible that mosquitoes laden with the micro-filaria may fall into water and perish, the filariæ being subsequently swallowed in water, or even that they may enter the skin in bathing.

Filariasis and the diseases produced by it only occur in tropical countries and even there are not serious as compared with ankylostomiasis or malaria; but the discovery of the life-history of filariæ has opened the way to the rapid diminution of malaria and the approaching extinction of yellow fever, as will be seen in Chapters XVII and XVIII.

### TEXAS FEVER

The story of Theobald Smith's investigation of the source of Texas Fever is as fascinating as that of Patrick Manson on filariasis, of Ronald Ross on malaria, or of Walter Reed and his colleagues on yellow fever; and it formed one of the chief initial links in the life-saving chain of tropical hygiene. A few dates will indicate the sequence of events. It is clear that investigators in the two hemispheres were consciously or unconsciously helped by the earlier or almost contemporaneous work of other investigators.

1872 The filaria *Sauguinis hominis* was found in blood by T. Lewis.

1876 Patrick Manson traced the life history of filariae found in human blood and in the mosquito.

1880 Laveran observed the malarial organisms in the blood of patients.

1893 Theobald Smith discovered the protozoon of Texas Fever.

1894 Manson published his hypothesis of mosquito carriage of malaria (*Pyrosoma bigeminum*).

1894 David Bruce proved that the tsetse fly (*Glossina morsitans*) spreads the *Trypanosoma brucei* from big game to cattle and horses.

1897 Ronald Ross traced the life cycle of malaria in birds.

1897–8 MacCallum and Opie demonstrated sexual conjugation in the flagella forms of the malarial plasmodium.

1899 H. R. Carter showed that a yellow fever patient cannot infect others until 10 to 14 days have elapsed since this patient was bit by a mosquito.

1900 Walter Reed and his colleagues proved the transmission of Yellow Fever by the *Stegomyia fasciata* (*Aedes calopus*).

Theobald Smith (born 1859) graduated as a physician; and at a time when Koch was being resorted to as the chief instructor in the technique of bacteriology, Smith obtained a post in the Bureau of National Industry at Washington. He studied and acquired skill in Koch's methods; and in 1888 he was set the definite task by his official chief of discovering the cause of Texas Fever, a disease of cattle, which was devastating the herds in many parts of America. Cattle were dying in large numbers when shipped East for beef; and apart from this much destruction occurred.

Theobald Smith's first investigations on current bacteriological lines failed; and then his helper Kilborne told him of the farmer's far-fetched but somewhat prevalent theory that the disease was carried by a tick which lived on and sucked the blood of the cattle.

Perhaps Smith's recollection that a similar story among dairy maids had led to Jenner's momentous discovery of vaccination against small pox, and that the source of malaria according to some was to be found in the bite of mosquitoes, may have had some influence in leading him to determine to investigate the tick theory. Whether so or not, in the next year 1889 he proceeded to experiment.

Smith and Kilborne in June of that year put several southern cattle infested with ticks along with an equal number of northern beasts free from ticks. Then three southern tick-infested cattle were taken, and all the ticks on them were picked off most laboriously and some healthy northern beasts were placed with them. The healthy cattle in the first experiment soon fell ill with Texas Fever, while in the second experiment they remained well!

Meanwhile, helped by Mr. Curtice, a Government expert in biology, the life-history of ticks was studied. They found that the immature ticks climb from the soil up the cow, acquire two additional legs—now having eight—suck the blood of the cow, then the females drop off the cow to deposit several thousands of eggs on the field.

On examination of the blood from the cattle which had died from Texas Fever in the above experiments, pear-shaped bodies were found in the blood and it was clear that these had devitalised the blood cells, and produced the characteristic symptoms of the disease. They were never found in healthy cattle.

Cattle did not acquire Texas fever when fed on hay containing infected ticks. So that ingestion was not the mode of infection.

Then a number of healthy cattle from the North were turned into the field where many cattle had died. These fell ill and died of Texas Fever. Evidently the grass of contaminated fields could convey the infected ticks to healthy cattle.

But if the contaminated field were left for 30 days before cattle were put in it, they did not become infected. To clear up this point, Smith began to breed ticks in his laboratory. These ticks are wood-lice, belonging to the acarines and closely related to the acarus which causes scabies. Young ticks thus bred from ticks like those which had spread Texas fever, when placed on healthy cattle produced the same fever. Evidently then the progeny of infected ticks could pass on the infection, and the explanation of the thirty days interval mentioned above was to be found in the time needed for the succession of generations to occur.

Theobald Smith's discovery was the pioneer discovery of the dual relation between a blood inhabiting and pathogenic protozoon (plasmodium) and an articulate or insect host and a mammalian host. It stands side by side in importance with the later work of Ross.

The way to prevent Texas Fever by depriving Southern cattle of their ticks by disinfectant "dips" was now clear, and a great economic gain was secured.

This investigation was almost contemporaneous with that of Sir David Bruce who proved the agency of the tsetse fly in carrying a trypanosome from big game to cattle and horses, and thus rendered possible measures for the prevention of tsetse-fly disease in these animals, and the vast economic loss associated with it.

Reference must be made to works on tropical medicine for the story of the further development of our knowledge of trypanosome diseases and the action thus rendered possible for the prevention of tropical "sleeping sickness."

# CHAPTER XVII

## The Prevention of Malaria

The history of malaria is one of slow diminution in many tropical countries, and of almost complete disappearance from countries with temperate climates, in which it formerly prevailed. Whether in Britain it has ever been continuously endemic is doubtful; but in recent centuries until about a hundred years ago it was not uncommon. The London Bills of Mortality returned many deaths each year from "fever and ague," and although some of these were not malaria, others were. The plays of Shakespeare, the diaries of Pepys and Evelyn show how prevalent ague was. James I and Charles II of England suffered from it. Cromwell died of a "quartan ague" and so did Evelyn's son. The reason for its disappearance will be better understood later; but it is significant that while an outbreak of malaria in the Thames estuary after the Crimean war apparently was associated with the return of troops from the Balkan peninsula, similar events in the Great War led to only a few indigenous cases of malaria in the civilian population, although anopheles were abundant.

In India in recent years malaria has caused many millions of deaths, and Rosenau states that in the South States of the United States there are a million cases of malaria every year.

The incidence of malaria varies greatly from year to year, presumably under the influence of varying temperature and humidity. New foci are occasionally established: thus the East African islands of Reunion and Mauritius were almost exempt until 1866 when a disastrous epidemic occurred. There is no doubt that, as in England, there were abundant anopheles in these islands; but, unlike in England, after the Great War, when many patients with malaria returned from the East, the other conditions in the above named islands which are indicated below favored the wide-spread of malaria.

Malaria until recent years has always been regarded as a soil-generated disease, especially of soil "the energies of which are not expended in growth and sustenance of healthy vegetation." All the earlier writings describe malaria as a "marsh miasm" or a "telluric poison." Malaria was responsible for the greater part of the sickness and mortality in many parts of the globe; and as Parkes put it, when a climate was described as "unhealthy," it simply meant it was malarious. Cases of malaria occurring elsewhere than in the vicinity of marshes were assumed to be due to a wind-blown miasm; water was also supposed to carry infection.

Apart from the more favored regions in which malaria diminished as populations became more urban and concentrated and as land drainage and cultivation extended, malaria has continued through the ages to be a source of decimation of populations, and enfeeblement of survivors. MacCulloch in 1872 traced its influence in causing race degeneration in various parts of the world, and W. H. S. Jones in 1909 (in *Malaria and Greek History*) concluded that malaria played a large part in bringing about the decadence of Greece.

So long as the above mentioned indefinite views of the causation of malaria prevailed, but little prevention was possible. Beauperthay, a French physician in the West Indies, in 1853 had argued that malaria was caused by mosquitoes, and A. F. A. King, a Washington physician had argued similarly in 1883, but without experimental testing of the hypothesis.

In 1880 Laveran, a French Army surgeon stationed at Algiers observed minute bodies in the red blood cells of malarious patients, which he regarded as a low form of animal life causing malaria. These bodies grew at the expense of the red cells, depositing a dark pigment; they assumed various forms including one called by Laveran "rosace." He thus saw various stages of the parasite, and as Ross states "from the first divined that the mosquito is connected with the propagation of these parasites." In 1889 Golgi of Pavia observed the differences between the rosaces or rosettes of tertian and quartan forms of malaria, found these to be constant, and concluded that they represented different species of organism. He ascertained also that the occurrence of fever coincided with the completion of the asexual cycle of the rosettes and the shedding of mesozoites into the blood. These attached themselves to or entered other blood cells and in two days in tertian and three days in quartan fever again completed another asexual cycle, with a geometrical increase in the possibilities of infection. Then a third species of parasite was recognized including crescentic bodies (gamocytes). This was found to be limited to the specially dangerous "aestivo-autumnal" form of malaria, and the physician thus was enabled by his microscope to realise the dangerous type of disease against which he was fighting.

How did the parasite gain access to the blood? Patrick Manson suggested that the flagellate forms of the plasmodium of malaria constituted a sporulating stage of the parasite, and that the agent for their distribution was a mosquito or "a similar suctorial insect." The fact that the Polymitus ("flagellate") stage was not found in the human body, but only developed *after the blood was drawn*, led him to regard the suctorial insect as the natural host at this stage of the life cycle of the plasmodium. He was unable to work at this hypothesis himself, being in England, but Sir Ronald (then Major) Ross of the Indian Medical Service while in England in 1894 was impressed by Manson's hypothesis and, keeping in touch with Manson at each stage of his investigation after returning to India in 1894, eventually demonstrated its accuracy. Bad luck for long months baffled Ross's search. He was in fact, investigating the wrong mosquito, and there were few cases of human malaria available for investigation in his station.

Manson suggested that Ross should work out the life history of the corresponding parasites in birds; and observations on these were completely successful. Ross's reports on Proteosoma, the malarial parasite of the sparrow, appeared in May and October, 1896. They established that the parasites in the blood cells of the sparrow are abstracted by a blood-sucking fly, subsequently identified as the *Culex fatigans.* He traced the bird parasite into the stomach of the mosquito, watched its growth, and its travel thence into the salivary gland, down the proboscis and back again into a bird, and measured the increase in size of the pigmented bodies at each stage. The stages of growth shown by the plasmodium in the culex demonstrated that two hosts were necessary for its complete life cycle, the culex thus being not merely a mechanical carrier of infection but also an obligate host.

In 1897 MacCallum (*Journal of Experimental Medicine*, January, 1898) found that, in Halteridium (Hœmoproteus) a blood parasite of birds closely analogous to the malarial parasite of man, the function of the flagellum is to impregnate certain free halteridia spheres, which when impregnated, as seen and described by him, assume an elongated shape (vermiculus) and accumulate characteristic pigment in their interior.

In 1899 Grassi and Bignami proved that human malaria is spread only by an anopheles mosquito. Grassi made an exhaustive research in Italy during 1898 to prove this point; and during the following winter his conclusion that an anopheles was the agent for transmitting human malaria was demonstrated by experiment on a human subject. This completed the proof of the method of infection of man. The general method of infection had been demonstrated by Ross's painstaking and persistent work, and his work and the forecast of Manson founded on his own prior work on filariasis manifest the characteristics of genius.

The experimental observations partially summarised in the preceding paragraphs amply justified Manson (*British Medical Journal*, June, 1898) in claiming that he could no longer justly be regarded as a sort of pathological Jules Verne, or as "guided by the divining rod of preconceived idea;" but that on the contrary the theory—it now rightly claimed this name rather than that of hypothesis—was the logical outcome of well-ascertained fact and the most promising guide for action. We may add the following quotations from the same article:

> Despite my critics, I still think that work undertaken with the object of advancing knowledge is most economically expended if directed by "speculative consideration" and "preconceived idea," provided these considerations and ideas are founded on facts, and are compatible with ascertained facts.

He concludes his remarks by the following summary:

> My object in making this communication is three-fold. First, again to call the attention of workers on malaria to this promising field of investigation; secondly, to place on record

Ross's claim to priority in discovery; and lastly, to vindicate myself from the charge of unscientific and unwarrantable speculation.

Manson had forecasted that different species of malarial parasite may require different kinds of mosquito as their alternative hosts, and this was verified by Ross's work and that of Grassi and others. Daniels identified the relatively rare mosquitoes with which Ross had succeeded in his human observations to be *Anopheles*, while the common fly which was concerned in the malaria of birds belonged to the genus *Culex*. Christophers and Stephens showed that in a native population in a malarious district a very high proportion of the children harbour malarial parasites in their blood.

Under Manson's guidance at a later stage two experiments were made with the definite object of demonstrating *coram publico* the pathogenesis of malaria. These experiments are described by Manson in *British Medical Journal*, September 29, 1900. He first referred in this article to the work of Grassi and Bignami who experimentally conveyed malaria to a man by the bite of mosquito. This experiment was possibly open to criticism, because it was performed in a malarial district. The two new experiments were free from this possible fallacy:

*A*. Relays of mosquitoes were arranged to be sent from Rome to London, the dispatch being expedited by special courtesy of the postal authorities. It was also provided that no infected mosquitoes carrying the malignant tertian parasites should be sent. The second consignment arrived with a fair proportion of the mosquitoes alive. Manson's son, aged 23, who had not been out of England since childhood was the subject on which 5 of these mosquitoes were fed by biting on August 29, 3 more on September 3, and large numbers on September 10 and 12. He developed an attack of typical malaria on the 13th September 1900, and in May the following year a relapse occurred.

*B.* A wooden hut constructed in England was erected in an intensely malarious part of the Roman Campagna where the inhabitants suffer from malarial cachexia. The hut was provided with fly-proof wire screened windows and doors. Drs. Sambon and Low and three others lived in this hut through a malarious season, took no quinine, and adopted no precaution except to keep indoors from sunset to sunrise. All of them escaped malaria.

Summarising the practical inferences from these two experiments Manson concluded:

> These experiments, together with the work of Ross, Grassi, Celli, Bignami, Bastianelli, and other Italians, the recent observations on native malaria by Koch, and the representatives of the Malaria Commission of the Royal Society and Colonial Office, plainly indicate that the practical solution of the malaria problem lies in
>
> 1. Avoiding the neighbourhood of native houses—the perennial source of malaria parasites.
>
> 2. The destruction, so far as practicable, of *Anopheles*' breeding pools.
>
> 3. And principally: Protection from mosquito bite.

He added

> The question of expense cannot for a moment be entertained in discussing the means for protection. One life saved, one invaliding obviated, would, even in a pecuniary sense, pay for all the wire gauze and mosquito netting requisite to protect every European house in West Africa.

In the same article he drew a moral which has significance for other great banes of mankind as for instance, tuberculosis, as well as for malaria. It is argued that one cannot avoid infection entirely. How then can measures against malaria be successful? The answer is that reduction of possibilities of infection minimises the risk.

In this connection Daniels has stated that in Central Africa not one mosquito in a thousand carries the malarial zygotes. Thus if he is bitten ten times every night, he is probably inoculated with malaria four times a year, whereas if protected at night and only bitten once a month he may not be infected in a hundred years!

In view of the life-history of the malarial plasmodium evidently many circumstances are concerned in the completion of its life-cycle, and therefore many measures may succeed in thwarting its personal and family history.

Whether malaria will or will not continue will depend on the factors enumerated by Ross and others in the following statement:

1. An accessible population.
2. The number of infected people in these.
3. The average number of these containing the sexual forms (sporozoites) of the parasite to infect anopheline mosquitoes.
4. The number of anopheles.
5. The number of anopheles feeding on a single person.
6. The proportion of these surviving a week.
7. The proportion of these survivors biting a human being.

Evidently failure of transmission may occur at any one of these stages. In England for instance the disappearance of the disease has been helped by the systematic use of quinine (preventing the development of sexual forms of the plasmodium), by the drainage of marshes, by the fact that in many seasons the conditions of temperature and moisture do not favor the life cycle of mosquitoes, by the fact that improved housing has diminished the harbouring of mosquitoes.

In Italy in 1923 only about 3000 deaths from malaria occurred, in the years 1887–1922 according to A. Castiglioni the number averaged 15,000 per annum. According to the same authority the chief factors concerned in this reduction had been the State distribution of quinine at low prices, the introduction of a rapidly breeding and larva-eating fish, the *Gambusia affinis*, into streams and ponds, and the increased breeding of cattle in malarious regions. Mosquitoes prefer cattle to human beings. This has probably been a factor in the disappearance of malaria from England. Chemical warfare against the larvae by spraying ponds is a valuable auxiliary. Mosquito nets for patients are important, as is also protective screening of all dwellings in malarious districts.

# CHAPTER XVIII

## The Prevention of Yellow Fever

The history of yellow fever prior to the discovery that it is mosquito-borne is full of tragedy. It occurred chiefly between latitudes 45° N. and 35° S., and its further spread was found to depend on the air temperature remaining as high as 70°F. It has been endemic in the West Indies and on the shores of the Gulf of Mexico, and more generally in tropical and sub-tropical regions, and it has generally appeared in and around ports, disappearing for instance in the highlands of Jamaica. It has been most fatal in crowded cities, especially ports; and long before its method of spread was ascertained, it was recognised that the congregation of persons born in a cold climate favoured its transmission; also that however violent was an epidemic it was arrested suddenly as soon as frost appeared. Negroes were regarded as immune, a condition now better explained by the occurrence of mild attacks in early life.

The extent of former prevalence in America may be exemplified by the experience of epidemic years in Philadelphia. Epidemics occurred in 1693, 1699, 1741, 1747, 1762, 1793–1794, 1797–1799, 1802–1805, 1819–1820, 1853, 1858. In this city in 1793 with 40,000 inhabitants 4,041 deaths from yellow fever occurred.

In Memphis in 1878, 5,750 deaths from yellow fever occurred.

In New Orleans in 1853, 8,101 deaths from yellow fever occurred.

In Lisbon in 1857 there were 13,757 known attacks and 5,625 deaths. In 1865 an outbreak in Britain occurred at Swansea. There were 70 cases and 50 deaths. Infection had been brought by a sailing vessel from Cuba. Previous small outbreaks had occurred in the same port in 1843, 1851, and 1864.

Various views have been held as to its causation. Prior to 1793 it was regarded as a divine visitation, then opinion wavered between the view that it was imported from the West Indies and the view that it was spontaneously generated under favoring conditions of filth and of atmospheric heat and moisture (see also page 134, *Evolution of Preventive Medicine*).

About 1878 fomites, intermediate infection by various articles, began to be regarded as important, and this view held good in administration until 1898–1899, rigid disinfection of places and of various articles being enforced.

Yellow fever illustrates perhaps better than any other disease how, without accurate knowledge of the natural history of a disease, humanity may flounder for decades or even centuries in helpless blundering; being dependent for protection during this period of darkness on the natural limitations to the spread of the disease afforded by climate and by infrequency of human communications.

Gradually enlightenment came, but in 1871 no mention was made of insect-borne disease in any standard medical work. Dr. J. Nott of Mobile, who introduced General Gorgas into the world in 1848, appears first to have attributed a part to insects in disseminating yellow fever (Nuttall "On the Rôle of Insects" in *Johns Hopkins Hospital Reports*, vol. viii), and he referred to the special danger at night.

Dr. C. J. Finlay (1835–1915) in 1881–1886 advanced similar views, and in 1891 he reported having subjected 67 persons to the bites of supposedly infected mosquitoes. His experiments were not conducted scientifically and he appears to have failed largely because having fed mosquitoes on yellow fever patients, he then fed these mosquitoes within 2 to 5 days on susceptible persons. It is noteworthy that he picked out the stegomyia mosquito from some 600 to 700 species as being the one which he regarded as the vector of yellow fever;. this was described by Gorgas as a great example of medical clairvoyance. It may be noted also that he supplied the eggs from which Walter Reed some years later reared his first experimental mosquitoes, with the brilliant success described below; and Reed in his account of his own work gave Finlay the credit for the mosquito theory. It may be added that Finlay planned the plan of campaign against yellow fever which followed on Reed's experimental results.

The main investigation which cleared up the problem of yellow fever was inspired by the investigations of Manson and Ross. Before describing it, we may outline the history of yellow fever in Havana, Cuba, as given by General Gorgas (*Lancet*, September 6, 1902).

In 1898 Colonel Waring had been sent to Havana, to "clean up" the city and to exterminate yellow fever, which for a century had been endemic in it. He succeeded in his sanitation, but next year an unusually severe outbreak of yellow fever occurred, especially in the better parts of the city.

The history of yellow fever in Havana in earlier years is shown in figure 7. The number of deaths had varied greatly, but each year they were numerous. In 1901 there were 18 deaths, in 1905 one case occurred; and then during the next eighteen years not a single case occurred (*Life and work of W. C. Gorgas*, 1924). During the years of yellow fever, the experience had been that it was limited almost entirely to foreigners.

Major Gorgas was appointed chief sanitary officer in Havana in 1898. For five years Havana had been the scene of military operations, and the city was "a great cesspool." Sanitary measures were rigorously pursued as indicated above, on the supposition that yellow fever was a filth disease; but notwithstanding these measures, including disinfection of premises on a large scale, yellow fever caused more deaths in 1900 than in 1898 (fig. 7). Yellow fever was so serious to the American troops that Havana might have had to be evacuated by them if the war with Spain had not ended speedily. The end of the Cuban war meant increased immigration of people. In 1900 25,000 arrived, chiefly from Spain, and this meant a "flare-up" of yellow fever, which occurred chiefly in the more sanitary districts.

In 1899 Dr. Henry R. Carter, published the results of important epidemiological researches on yellow fever carried on for several years in the Mississippi valley. He found on tabulating dates of exposure and attack of those acquiring yellow fever in isolated farm houses that persons who visited these houses during the 10 to 14 days following the date of onset of the first patient's attack did not contract the disease; but that later visitors became ill; also that the infected house was dangerous after the patient's death or removal. Carter ascertained that the incubation period of yellow fever was five days, but that as indicated above a two or three weeks interval elapsed before the house occupied by a yellow fever patient became infected. Clearly then the patient himself was not the direct source of infection, but his environment.

Walter Reed at this time was a member of the medical staff of the American Public Health Service, and General Wood was the Military Governor of Cuba. He happily also was a man who had received medical training. It was not difficult, therefore, to prove the desirability of pursuing in the case of yellow fever an investigation which would extend the discoveries already made by Manson and Ross and by Theobald Smith, and which would, furthermore, demonstrate whether the conclusion deducible from Carter's epidemiological investigations was correct, —namely, that the interval between primary and secondary cases of yellow fever implied a stage in the development of an infective agent in some insect host.

In 1900 a Commission was appointed, on the initiation of Dr. G. M. Sternberg, the Surgeon General of the American Army, composed of Drs. Reed, Carroll and Lazear, with the subsequent addition of Dr. A. Agramonte, to investigate yellow fever in Cuba. The investigation was one for finding the method of spread, not for discovering the specific microbe causing yellow fever. More recently Noguchi has isolated a spirochæte from the blood of yellow fever patients, which is only found in the first three days of the attack.*

Reed and his colleagues disproved the infectiousness of fomites. Volunteer soldiers slept with impunity on beds recently vacated by yellow fever patients, and in close contact with soiled linen from these patients; though the same soldiers when allowed to be bitten by the common house mosquito of tropical America, *Stegomyia fasciata*, now known as the *Aedes calopus*, developed yellow fever.

Lazear and Carroll inoculated themselves with mosquitoes which had bitten yellow fever patients, without result. They had been bitten by stegomyias not fulfilling the conditions of Carter's discovery as to "extrinsic incubation"—the interval which transpires

*See postscript, page 163.

in the biting mosquito before it becomes infective. Subsequently these investigators were bitten again experimentally and both were attacked, Lazear's attack being fatal. American soldiers volunteered for further experiments. In the course of experiments on them it was found that those having had a previous attack of yellow fever were immune; and that non-immunes under no circumstances acquired the disease unless bitten by an infected mosquito. Furthermore it was learnt that the mosquito in order to become infected must bite the yellow fever patient during the first three days of his illness; and the experiments on soldiers confirmed Carter's finding that the infected mosquito is harmless for 10 to 14 days after it has bitten a patient.

The stegomyia which was proved to be the special vector of yellow fever has been known for centuries as a house-dweller, common in cities. It breeds in or about houses, and has been called also the "cistern mosquito." In this connection may be mentioned the experience of New Orleans in which notwithstanding vast improvements, yellow fever recurred at intervals until its many thousands of domestic water-butts were abolished or securely sealed.

The stegomyia has been found to remain infective at the end of 57 days, and it is stated that infectivity may persist for five months.

The facts revealed in this splendid investigation by Reed and his associates have been followed by preventive work which has almost removed yellow fever from the face of the earth. The first demonstration was in Cuba, with the striking results shown in figure 7. There followed the construction of the

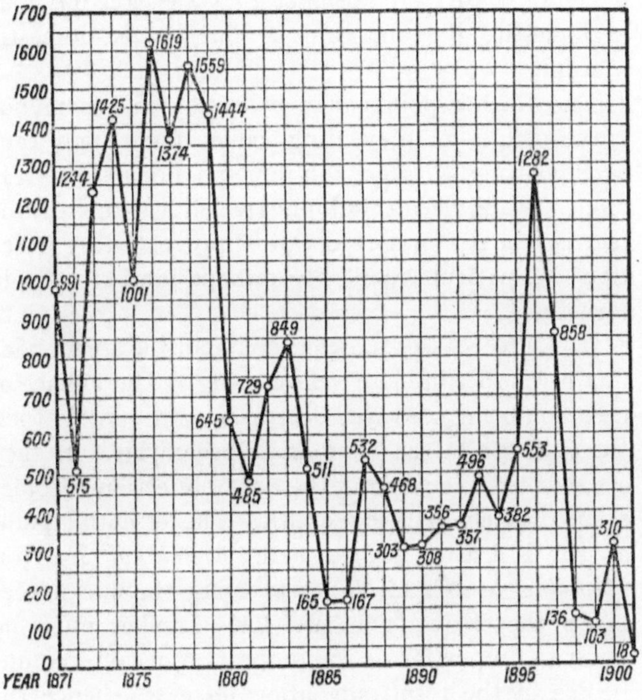


FIG. 7. EXPERIENCE OF YELLOW FEVER IN CUBA

Panama Canal, which was rendered practicable by the anti-malarial and anti-yellow-fever work organized under Gorgas' leadership. This story is well known. It formed the greatest administrative triumph of tropical preventive medicine. Anti-malarial measures coincide with those against yellow fever, with the exception of treatment by quinine, and the difference in action based on the fact that the stegomyia is a domestic, the anopheles a chiefly non-domestic breeder.

Two further points may be noted. Is there not grave danger in preventing yellow fever, and thus accumulating a large non-immune population? If modern public health administration is adopted, this fear is a bogy; for spread can be prevented by isolation of patients and by prompt anti-stegomyia measures.

It is unnecessary to exterminate all the stegomyias in a town to eliminate yellow fever. The chance of infection being conveyed decreases more rapidly than the decrease in the number of stegomyias. If they are reduced to one-third, the risk of infection becomes approximately only one-ninth. The essential point as H. R. Carter pointed out (*Annals of Tropical Medicine*, March 15, 20) is to bring the mosquitoes below the critical number. This number must be fewer in proportion as the proportion of non-immune people in the total population increases; hence the importance of early recognition of cases, and the need to remember that non-reporting of cases does not of itself imply their non-existence.

In view of the fact that one attack of yellow fever—unlike malaria—immunises against second attacks, a community in the tropics may free itself from yellow fever while doing nothing to this end. Danger begins to recur when non-immune persons are introduced into the community by birth or by immigration. But in modern circumstances of life it is evident that the only method of safety against yellow fever consists in the prompt detection and isolation (from mosquitoes) of every case of the disease, and the steady persistence in extermination of stegomyias in and about houses, and in abolition of all receptacles in which they can breed.

*Postscript.* Investigation in West Africa during 1928 has shown that Noguchi's spirochete is not the cause of yellow fever. Stokes and his co-workers have shown that it is due to a filter-passing virus. Noguchi while bravely testing this new work, fell a victim to yellow fever as did also Stokes and the physician attending Noguchi. More recently Dr. Sellards of Harvard University has brought this virus to London, where Dr. Hindle, working on the basis of successful work on dog distemper virus by Dr. Laidlow, and of similar work on fowl plague virus by Dr. C. Todd, has proved that susceptible monkeys can be protected against yellow fever by suitable vaccination. Similar vaccination will probably be successful for man (see Sir W. Fletcher's letter, *Times*, November 18, 1928).

## CHAPTER XIX

### The Prevention of Venereal Diseases

The two diseases syphilis and tuberculosis,—both running in the majority of cases a course protracted over many years—are responsible for a large share of the total deaths of mankind which occur before old age. In some years of adult life tuberculosis still causes half of all deaths that occur. The deaths from syphilis are incompletely stated in the returns of death registration; but if the later effects of this disease, direct and indirect, are included, there can be little doubt that it ranks among the four or five chief agents of death occurring before old age is reached.

We need not attempt to decide whether in this respect tuberculosis, syphilis, cancer or pneumonia is the most serious; though, if we look at life as an opportunity for repaying the debt incurred in our rearing and adolescence, the two first named must be placed first in importance, as producing the greatest amount of invalidity and mortality before life's accumulated owings have been repaid by life's work.

Syphilis is the major venereal disease. Like gonorrhoea, in the adult it is almost entirely traceable to impure sex relationships; and if we recall that these diseases in children, in innocent wives and in others acquired by accident, were originally produced as the result of earlier sexual promiscuity, the statement can stand without exception.

Syphilis is a frequent cause of still-births and of premature live-birth of diseased infants. It is a frequent cause of death in infancy and childhood. It is often responsible for partial blindness, and for deafness which may appear to be hereditary. Acquired in early manhood, it is a chief agent of premature arterial degeneration. It is responsible for practically all deaths from aortic aneurism, and for a high proportion of the deaths from cerebral hœmorrhage, especially those occurring in middle life. General paresis of the insane, the disease from which some 15 to 20 per cent of the patients admitted to mental asylums are suffering, is due solely to the syphilitic virus. Scarcely an organ of the body escapes attack by the virus of syphilis, and the toll of mischief wrought by it is immensely greater than is generally known.

Gonorrhoea is commonly regarded as a not very serious disease; but this is erroneous. In infants infection with the gonococcus at birth causes an acute ophthalmia which is responsible for some 30 to 40 per cent of the inmates of blind asylums. Gonorrhoea is the chief cause of involuntary sterility in women, and in more than half the women infected by it there is said to occur inflammation of the female pelvic organs, often leading to chronic invalidity. The gonococcus not infrequently causes gonococcal infection of the heart. In both syphilis and gonorrhoea infectivity is very prolonged, especially if treatment is neglected.

The history of these two banes of humanity is an important element in the social history of mankind. Gonorrhoea doubtless is a very ancient disease. As to the origin of syphilis there is much dispute. Ancient writings do not throw much light. There appears to be no satisfactory evidence of syphilitic lesions in ancient bones or mummies; but the retroussé nose with a defective bridge shown in apparently genuine pictures of Socrates and of Augustus Caesar have been quoted as evidence of syphilis. The absence of definite evidence of syphilis is not conclusive; for, as Sudhoff says (*Essays in the History of Medicine*, by Sudhoff, translated by Garrison and others, 1926): "in the field of infectious diseases, ancient medicine suffered from marked weakness of vision." There is similar lack of evidence of syphilis in pre-Columbus days in America. Dr. Hrdlička, working for the Smithsonian Institution, has concluded from examination of some hundred skeletons that no sure sign of syphilis prior to Columbus has been found in the New World; though abundant evidence of the ravages of syphilis is found in skeletons in Indians graves of the seventeenth and eighteenth centuries. But Dr. Hayhurst of Ohio University in 1927 quotes Dr. Means who from radiographic work has concluded that there is gross evidence of syphilis in the skeletons of Mounds, offshooots of the ancient Maya civilization of Central America (*British Medical*

*Journal*, 1927). Hirsch concluded that confusion between syphilis and leprosy was responsible for the statement that the movements of Crusaders caused a wide spread of leprosy. Whether this be so or not, it is not even certain that the terrible European epidemic of "syphilis" in the fifteenth century was entirely this disease. Sudhoff concludes that the epidemic at Naples, among the invading troops of Charles VIII of France, was really typhoid or paratyphoid fever. The dispersal of the mercenary troops of this monarch were regarded as responsible for dispersing the "Morbus Gallicus" over Italy. These troops had been in Italy from September, 1494; while Columbus had arrived back from Hayti in the West Indies at Barcelona in April, 1493. But it remains doubtful whether his sailors were the vectors of a "new" infection to the French troops and their camp followers. The stars were blamed for the new disease; also a general corruption of the air, especially as nurses and priests were attacked. For the latter especially, infection by aerial convection was invoked. Baümler in Ziemssen's *Cyclopedia*, vol. iii, maintains that the disease existed in Spain before Charles VIII's campaign, and before the return of Columbus. On the contrary Jonathan Hutchinson has urged that if syphilis had been known in Europe before 1492 it would have been mentioned by Chaucer and Boccaccio. General circumstances, including a succession of bad seasons and famine in France and Germany 1491–1495, along with the vast military operations, doubtless helped to render this first known great epidemic of syphilis excessively serious.

So late as 1787 John Hunter inoculated himself with pus which he thought to be solely gonorrhoeal and produced syphilis, which shortened his days. From this experiment, and partly also because he held the erroneous view that one could only suffer from one infection at a time, he concluded that gonorrhoea and syphilis are caused by the same poison. Their separate identity was only settled definitely by numerous inoculations made by Ricord (1799–1889). His treatise on venereal disease was published in 1838.

Gradually syphilis became less virulent in its earlier lesions. These have become markedly less serious even during the last 70 years, but it is doubtful whether this denotes in part an attenuated virus, or is chiefly the result of greater cleanliness in treatment of wounds and in the earlier adoption of satisfactory specific treatment.

That even as early as 1494 syphilis was seriously regarded in many countries is indicated by the following regulation dated April 21, 1497 (made into rather more modern English), which is quoted from Dr. J. D. Crombie's *History of Scottish Medicine*, 1927.

It was ordained by the aldermen and council for the avoidance of the infirmity come out of France and strange parts, that all light women be charged and ordered to desist from their vices of sin and venery, and all their houses emptied, and that they work for their sustentation, under the pain of a key of hot iron on their cheeks and banishment from the town.

Modern knowledge of syphilis has greatly increased the possibilities of controlling it. In the year 1903 Metschnikoff and Roux transmitted the disease to monkeys and demonstrated the prophylactic value of calomel inunctions. Earlier inoculations appeared to show that most monkeys are immune to syphilis, but these investigators found that in the chimpanzee primary and secondary lesions like those of man are produced after inoculation. (See four communications in *Annales de l'Institut Pasteur*, beginning December, 1903.) A chimpanzee was inoculated over the eyebrow with virus from the hard chancres of two men; then three-quarters of an hour later the part was rubbed for ten minutes with an ointment containing equal parts of mercury and of benzoated lard. No syphilitic lesion followed; but a control chimpanzee similarly inoculated developed syphilis; and the first chimpanzee when later on inoculated with syphilitic virus developed syphilis.

Similar experiments with calomel produced protection without the local irritating effect of metallic mercury.

In 1905 Schaudinn discovered the protozoon or spirochœte in primary lesions of syphilis and in 1911 Noguchi cultivated this (*Spir. pallida*) in artificial culture. In 1913 he elucidated the true nature of general paresis of the insane and of locomotor ataxy (tabes dorsalis) by discovering this spirochœte in the brain and spinal cord respectively.

In 1906 Wassermann, Neisser and Bruck introduced the serological test, enabling a correct diagnosis to be made when clinical evidence of syphilis is dubious.

Evidently the above enumerated discoveries gave increased accuracy to the diagnosis of the primary lesions (by discovery of the spirochœte) and to the diagnosis of later lesions by the Wassermann reaction; while the application of calomel ointment at the time of or shortly after exposure to infection greatly diminishes the risk of inoculation of the disease.

A further and most important step in control of syphilis was made by Ehrlich (1854–1915) to whose life-work special reference may be made here. His life story is a romance in organic chemistry. In his earlier studies he showed that animal tissues could be stained differentially by anilin dyes, and thus was made possible advance in modern bacteriology. In 1890–1899 in the course of his investigation of toxins and antitoxins as bearing on immunity in infectious diseases, he evolved his side-chain theory. From 1899–1906 his studies of hœmolysins led to the development of the theory of ambiceptors, with which his side-chain theory was completed. This work and the prior study of antibodies by Bordet and Gengou led to the discovery of the Wassermann test for syphilis.

As early as 1902 Laveran and Mesnil found that in a disease of mice caused by trypanosomes (protozoal unicellular animal organisms), the administration of $As_2O_3$ (arsenious oxide) abated the disease without hurting the mice, but that deadly doses were required to prevent relapses. This led to assiduous search for harmless arsenical compounds which would attack trypanosomes or spirochœtes without injuring their host.

Koch cured tropical sleeping sickness by the administration of atoxyl, which had been introduced by Thomas of Liverpool in 1905.

In 1907 Ehrlich and his pupils found that in the treatment of sleeping sickness the trypanosomes may become resistant to atoxyl. A large number of other arsenical organic compounds were examined experimentally during four years, and after many attempts Ehrlich produced salvarsan (606) which when intravenously injected casuses rapid disappearance of syphilitic lesions, while the spirochœtes in superficial lesions are found to be dead. This immediate disinfecting effect of salvarsan has great public health importance.

In securing this great triumph in therapeutic and preventive medicine Ehrlich had been guided by the leading idea embodied in his side-chain theory, that chemical substances whether foods or drugs or poisons only act as such when they become chemically fixed to the cells or protoplasm upon which their specific action is exerted: that, in his own words, "corpora non agunt nisi fixata." The investigation of the structure of crystals by Pasteur seemed remote from the successful inoculation against hydrophobia, and it seemed equally far from Ehrlich's staining of leucocytes by anilin dyes to the production of salvarsan. In both instances success was achieved by steady pursuit of experimentation guided by genius.

The discovery of 606 by Ehrlich meant more than the control (and almost cure) of syphilis and invaluable aid in presenting its further dissemination. Other spirochœtal diseases yield to similar specific medication. The discovery of this drug realised the dream of the medicœval Paracelsus, who preached a new era in Chemistry, Yatro-chemistry, Chemistry in the service of man. Its discovery opened a vista of possible extension of preventive medicine by treatment. Whether it will ever be possible to kill the bacteria of acute infectious diseases and of tuberculosis remains to be seen, but pathogenic bacteria show differential staining by anilin dyes and the possibility is not entirely beyond belief.

It is clear from the preceding review that on its scientific side syphilis is entirely controllable because of the following known facts:

*a.* The existence of the disease, when clinically obscure, can be recognised by detection of the spirochœtes and later by the Wassermann test.

*b.* The phenomena of the disease can be suppressed, even if sometimes not all the spirochœtes in the system are killed, by specific treatment.

*c.* The local application of a preparation containing 30 per cent of calomel within an hour of exposure to infection suffices in most instances to prevent the spirochœtes from entering the system.

Action on these lines, especially on the first two, is being taken on a national scale in Great Britain, and there is evidence of a striking decrease in the death-rate from syphilis. Doubtless, however, a share of this decrease is owing to other factors, including a wide dissemination of knowledge of sex hygiene, and it may be hoped, also, an increasing realisation by each adolescent and adult that it is his duty to himself, to his future spouse, to his children hereafter to be born, and to the community of which he forms a unit, to pass on the flame of life untarnished by irregular and anti-social sex relationships.

The consideration of this supremely important part of the hygiene and ethics of sex cannot be undertaken here; but those further interested in this most fundamental of the problems of preventive medicine will find it more adequately stated in several chapters of my *Health Problems in Organised Society* (P. S. King and Son, 1927).

# CHAPTER XX

## The Prevention of Tuberculosis

Although much less fatal than in the past, human tuberculosis is still one of the chief causes of premature death, of chronic invalidism, and of social dependence in survivors of its victims.

Its place among the registered causes of death has already been shown in figure 1 on page 7. A further important point is elucidated by figure 8—comparison of the age incidence of deaths from tuberculosis and cancer. It will be seen that tuberculosis has killed about 97 per cent of its total victims before the age of 65 is reached, while at the same age cancer has only killed 60 per cent of its total victims. Both diseases are terribly serious socially and economically, as each of them is the cause of death of more than half of its victims during the working years of life—20 to 65.

The experience of the last 60 years has been one of great and steady decline in the death rate from tuberculosis. Thus in England and Wales in 1871–1875 the average death rate from Pulmonary Tuberculosis (Phthisis or Consumption) was 2.22, in 1924 it was 0.84 per 1000 of population, showing a decline of 62 per cent.

How has this decline been brought about? Is it the result of natural causes of unknown character, or can it be traced to human activities? A review of the history and the natural history of tuberculosis is necessary, before attempting to answer this question.

Hippocrates (460–377 B.C.) described a suppuration of the lungs, probably phthisis. Galen (130–200 A.D.) believed phthisis to be very infectious,

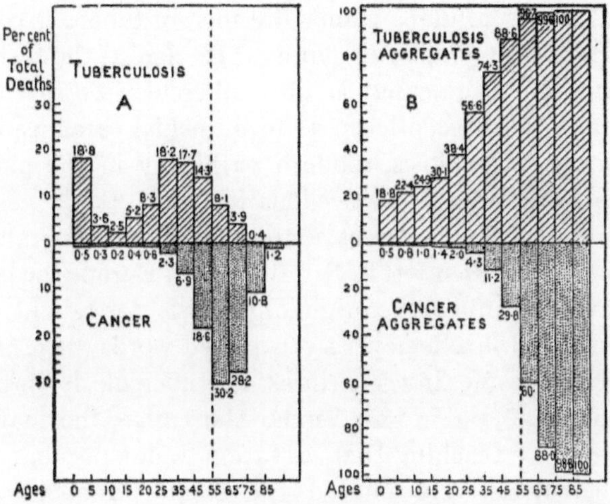


FIG. 8

while Avicenna (A.D. 1037) referred to "many diseases which are taken from man to man, like phthisis." The characteristic tuberculous nodules and their part in phthisis were described by F. D. Sylvius, (1614–1672) who regarded the nodules as lymphatic glands of the lungs. Morton in 1689 said that the tubercle is the pathological evidence of phthisis, and G. L. Bayle (1774–1816), the precursor of Laennec, traced minute tubercles through the subsequent stages of suppuration and caseation.

The investigations of Laennec (1781–1826) formed a veritable *tour de force* of objective analysis. He taught that every phthisis develops from tubercles, and that scrofulous glands are merely tubercles confined to the lymphatic glands. He denied the transformation of pneumonia into tuberculosis. In this, as also in his scepticism as to bronchial catarrh producing tuberculosis, modern pathology in the main has confirmed his marvellous insight.

Laennec's views were adopted by Louis in France and Hughes Bennett in Britain, but in Europe the primarily inflammatory origin of phthisis was taught, as illustrated in Niemeyer's oft-quoted words (page 18).

Microscopic investigations of tuberculosis began about 1840, and in 1847 Virchow buttressed the dualist theory by teaching that caseation is not peculiar to tuberculosis. He limited the term "tubercle" to miliary tubercle. In 1857 Buhl showed that in nine-tenths at least of cases of phthisis, caseous masses were pre-existent in some parts of the body, and he regarded tuberculosis as a sort of metastasis from these primary masses, an important step forward.

Experimental investigation brought further light. Klenke in 1843 injected tuberculous matter into the jugular vein of a rabbit, and six months later found tuberculosis of the liver and lungs.

Villemin's epoch-making results were published on December 5, 1865. He demonstrated the specificity of tuberculosis by injecting tuberculous material from a case of phthisis subcutaneously behind the ear of a healthy rabbit. Tubercular nodes developed; but no such nodes developed when non-tuberculous matter was inoculated. Villemin summed up his conclusions, derived from a number of experiments, of which one is cited above, as follows:

1. Tuberculosis is the effect of a specific causal agent, in short of a virus.
2. This agent must reside like its congeners in the morbid products formed by its direct action on the normal elements of the affected tissues.
3. Introduced into an organism susceptible of its action, it must continue to reproduce itself, and at the same time to reproduce the disease of which it is the essential principle and the determining cause. Experiment has confirmed these results of induction.

He added in summary: "tuberculosis is a specific affection, caused by an inoculable agent."

To Villemin belongs the honor of first distinguishing between the virus causing the disease and the lesions produced by it. His work was confirmed in 1868 by Burdon Sanderson in England. Sanderson also gave experimental evidence which was inconsistent with experiments made by others appearing to show that tuberculosis might result from inoculation of non-tuberculous material.

Cohnheim in 1880 inoculated tuberculous matter

into the anterior eye chamber of animals, and thus could watch each stage of tuberculosis of the iris and cornea.

On the basis of these results it became possible to prophesy the early discovery of the parasitic agent of tuberculosis, the final test of the accuracy of the sound induction already made. Prior to this discovery confirmation was given by repeated inoculations in various animals, and by Chauveau's experiments showing that tuberculosis could be produced by the eating of tuberculous meat.

There followed Pasteur's pioneer work, the introduction of Koch's improved technique, and the use of basic aniline dyes for staining bacteria. On March 24, 1882, Koch contributed to the Physiological Society of Berlin his note on "The Discovery and Cultivation of the Bacillus of Tuberculosis." He showed how the difficulty of demonstrating the specific *Bacillus tuberculosis* in tuberculous tissues had been overcome; how, while these remained unaffected by a watery solution of a basic aniline dye, they were stained by prolonged immersion in a solution of methylene blue to which potash had been added. The tubercle bacillus has a very resistant outer membrane to penetrate which this use of an alkali is required. It has been found also that while other stained bacilli are decolorized in a strong acid solution, the tubercle bacillus stained as above retains its color—a valuable diagnostic feature.

Koch overcame the further difficulty that the tubercle bacilli could not be cultivated in the artificial laboratory media hitherto employed. He inoculated the surface of solidified blood serum with tuberculous material. On this no growth occurred for ten days or more, but then a slow growth of tubercle bacilli began. It thus became possible to prove the specificity of the tubercle bacillus by following it through the stages demanded in Koch's postulates (page 43).

But although it is an axiomatic truth that in the absence of tubercle bacilli no tuberculosis occurs, and that the prevention of infection or at least the diminution of frequency and of dosage of infection is the primary object of preventive medicine as applied to tuberculosis, it is none the less essential to know all the circumstances favoring or impeding the life-history of the tubercle bacillus, and to utilise this knowledge by the adoption of indirect as well as of direct preventive measures. Strauss has defined tuberculosis as "a general disease characterised by miliary eruptions in the various organs"; and corresponding to varying dosage of infection, to differences of point of entry of infection and differences in acquired or intrinsic resistance to infection, there will occur either general or localised disease, an acute fatal disease or a local focus or foci which become encapsulated, and with favorable conditions of subsequent life, remain obsolescent.

With the discovery of the tubercle bacillus the initial tendency was to lay sole stress on infection. Even before Koch's discovery this view had received wide acceptance. In 1750 the articles and bedding belonging to consumptives were burnt in Nancy. In 1782 an edict in Naples ordered the isolation of consumptives and the disinfection of their belongings. In 1839 George Sand travelling in Spain with the consumptive Chopin was turned out of her hotel, and payment was demanded for the bed on which Chopin had slept. William Budd (*Lancet*, vol. ii, 1867, p. 451) propounded the theory that phthisis is a true zymotic disease, propagated by tuberculous matter from person to person: and he urged that by destroying this matter on its issue from the body and by auxiliary good sanitary conditions, we could hope to end this fatal scourge.

Experiments on animals have shown that tuberculosis can be communicated, not only by its inoculation, but also by inhalation or by ingestion. Guinea pigs acquire the disease if made to breathe air containing dust contaminated by tubercle bacilli; and various animals can be infected with tuberculosis by feeding them on the milk given by tuberculous cows. Pigs readily acquire infection in this way. Meat with tuberculous nodules on it has similarly given tuberculosis to various animals, and this possibility may not be obviated by imperfect cooking. It is unnecessary to detail the many experiments made to determine the relative infectivity of dried dust derived from the sputum of consumptives and the droplets of infective material ejected by consumptives when coughing. Both dangers exist, but in ordinary domestic life it is likely that the greatest risk is that arising from droplet infection. The dirt of rooms occupied by consumptive patients occasionally is found to contain tubercle bacilli, and uncleanliness is a great promoter of tuberculosis; but it is probable that even greater risk, especially for children, attaches to the soiled hands of consumptive patients after expectoration and to their fondling of children, without washing hands and without carefully screening the mouth during the act of coughing. Children in the crawling stage are particularly prone to be infected through their toys or from the floor, contaminated by careless patients.

In 1894 Ransome and Delepine proved that a two days' exposure to air and light with only one hour's sunshine sufficed to destroy the virulence of tuberculous sputum when it was exposed in a clean well lighted house. At that time great importance was attached to the long survival of tubercle bacilli in rooms of houses; but while this risk is one to be avoided by domestic cleansing, the tubercle bacillus is a true parasite, it does not multiply at ordinary temperatures of the external air, and it can only be cultivated artificially at or near the body temperature.

Even those who suffer from open tuberculosis are harmless so long as the tubercle bacilli expelled by them are prevented by cleanliness and careful precautions from infecting others. The patient becomes dangerous only when he is personally uncleanly, especially when he becomes so helpless that he can no longer see to the suitable ejection and disposal of his sputum. For the healthy the danger of infection increases in crowded rooms, and quite specially when these are also badly ventilated and inadequately lighted.

Tuberculosis very accurately has been described as a bedroom disease, for it is in circumstances of close and repeated intimacy that it chiefly spreads. The significance of such infection is often overlooked, because,—unless massive infection has occurred—the primary foci of disease become encapsulated, though liable to be released if subsequent conditions of life are unsatisfactory. Of such circumstances industrial life, especially the inhalation of dust stands first; but an attack of influenza or measles or some other infectious disease may act similarly, and the influence of alcoholic excess in "making the bed for tuberculosis" is well known.

In the past tuberculosis has caused a higher death rate in childhood than in adult life (i.e., per 1000 living at each age period). This death rate has declined at all ages, but much more in childhood than in adult life; and after allowing for possible changes in certification of death the statistics confirm experience in concluding that young children are now less exposed to infection and are exposed to infection in smaller doses than in past years. This special experience of childhood is consistent with converging lines of evidence that sanatoriums and hospital treatment of adult cases, the education of these adults in the hygienic management of their life, along with more adequate precautions in all cases of tuberculosis, are saving the lives of vast numbers of children and adolescents.

The influence of occupation on the amount of phthisis was emphasised by Dr. Headlam Greenhow in 1858 in reports to the English Privy Council. He showed that in proportion as people were attracted to indoor occupations, so this disease increased.

Dr. McCormack of Belfast in 1855 said:

> In a cosy room the consumptive is bound never to live, nor in any room, indeed, for great lengths of time. So long as he is able to be out of doors, he is in his best and safest home.
>
> Wherever there is foul air . . . . there we meet consumption, we meet scrofula, and an untimely death.

In 1858 a Commission was appointed to inquire into the sanitary state of the British Army. They concluded that the excess of phthisis in the Army was due mainly to "bad ventilation and the imperfect drainage of the barracks."

Poverty is associated with an excess of tuberculosis. The circumstances of this association are complex. They may include malnutrition, overwork, industrial dust, overcrowding, as well as increased direct infection. Koch is clear in his statement of the relative importance of these factors. He says:

> If one investigates more closely one finds that it is not poverty *per se* that favors tuberculosis, but the bad domestic conditions under which the poor everywhere, but especially in

great cities, have to live. . . . . It is the overcrowded dwellings of the poor that we have to regard as the real breeding places of tuberculosis.

During the Great War, especially in Central Europe, the mortality from tuberculosis greatly increased, and this has been commonly attributed to defective nutrition of the populations affected. This is going ahead of the facts. In peace times phthisis, in different countries, has not consistently followed the course of nutrition of populations. With malnutrition,—sometimes without it—go domestic overcrowding, dirty habits as to coughing and expectoration, and lack of hospital beds for acutely infectious cases. It is the almost inevitable result of an imperfect survey of events to attach undue importance to one among several contributory factors producing an evil result.

A considerable proportion of the tuberculosis in young children, especially of its non-fatal forms is due to infection by tubercle bacilli from cows' milk. Theobald Smith showed that the tubercle bacilli of bovine origin are thicker, shorter and more regular in shape than tubercle bacilli of human origin; also that they are dysgonic, i.e., show a scantier growth on various media than do the human type, which are hence called eugonic. He also showed that bovine tubercle bacilli are much more highly virulent for guinea pigs, rabbits and other animals than human tubercle bacilli, and that the inoculation of the latter into oxen produces only limited local lesions or no result.

But at the International Congress on Tuberculosis, 1901, held in London, Koch threw doubt on the possibility of bovine bacilli being, more than to a negligible extent, the cause of human disease. This led to further extensive investigation, the general effect of which was to confirm Theobald Smith's conclusions, to show that bovine infection is responsible for much disease in children, especially of glands and bones, and that there is no evidence of transfer of bovine into human type or vice versa.

Koch's scepticism undoubtedly was useful in bringing infection of bovine source into its correct less serious position in relation to infection of human source; but it did not justify failure to protect children against infected milk. It has been found that tubercle bacilli in milk are destroyed at 60°C. (140°F), and it is easy therefore to protect against this risk domestically or by commercial pasteurization of milk adequately controlled. The wider measures now being taken to protect the public by inspection of cattle and elimination of those giving tuberculous milk, the use of the tuberculin test, and systematized pasteurization of milk need not be detailed here.

Allusion has already been made to the importance of dosage in determining the extent and character of resulting tuberculosis. In experimental investigations it has been found that the larger the dose of bacilli injected into an animal of a given age and weight the greater the effect produced; and the larger the dose administered by feeding the more likely is infection to be caused.

The following comments are quoted from my annual report as Medical Officer to the Local Government Board, 1911–1912.

> The question of dosage of infection in tuberculosis has importance in view of the statements as to the ubiquity of the tubercle bacillus, on which has been based the assumption that measures increasing inherited or acquired resistance are more important than measures directed towards preventing massive infection. All investigations into the presence of tubercle bacilli in various places agree in showing that tubercle bacilli are found chiefly in the immediate environment of patients with open tuberculosis. A very high proportion of the population have received infection, and may have developed small nodules of disease, and will afterwards give positive tuberculin reactions, although the vast majority of them never have suffered or will suffer from clinically recognisable tuberculosis. Such "tuberculisation" for practical purposes needs to be distinguished from tuberculosis. The two conditions, doubtless, shade into one another, and the foci of tuberculisation may, under the provocation of an acute fever, such as measles or influenza, or of prolonged devitalising influences, become the center from which active disease develops. But observations on the incidence of tuberculosis in families point to the conclusion that the danger of effective infection is greatest under circumstances of protracted or repeated exposure to infection, especially when resistance is lowered by such influences as injury to the lungs by irritating dust, alcoholism, intercurrent illness, or privation.

This distinction between tuberculisation and tuberculosis is most important. It is likely that in persons specially susceptible, whether temporarily or permanently, a dosage of infection which in others would be harmless may excite active disease; but that in most instances so-called personal differences mean differences in amount of infective material acquired. There is more tuberculosis probably in the first year after birth than at any subsequent age, though this early tuberculosis is decreasing. For its further reduction removal of infants and young children from homes where the father or mother is consumptive has been practised. In most countries removal of the parent and his training in a hygienic life have been found more generally practicable.

Tested by the tuberculin test some 15 to 20 per cent of children under 3 years of age have been ascertained to be infected. Between the 3rd and 4th year of life 40 to 70 per cent respond positively to the cutaneous tuberculin test.

The question has been much debated as to whether this reception of tubercle bacilli in early life without the development of disease is to be regarded as partially vaccinal in character, which is probable; and whether when phthisis develops in adult life this is due to resuscitation of infective material received in early life or is caused by more recent infection in industrial life or otherwise. Almost certainly both suggestions are true; but it would be unwise to assume that disease the result of adolescent or adult infection occurs only exceptionally. The practical point at all ages is to prevent infection, or short of this to ensure such conduct on the part of all persons with cough and expectoration as will render infection except in minimal doses an unlikely event.

A further controversial point is as to whether a gradual process of immunization has been taking place in white races under civilized conditions. The civilized races recently exposed to infection undoubtedly suffer from excessively acute and severe tuberculosis. In this respect they resemble infants in civilized communities who are exposed to massive infection. In both instances no immunity has been previously established by prior exposure to lesser degrees of infection. It may be that some of the excessive tuberculosis in savage races in touch with civilized man represents greater susceptibility; but if so, there is doubtless also, owing to overcowding and dirty personal habits, an exceptionally heavy dosage of infection.

The modern outlook on tuberculosis is rightly optimistic. The course of the death rate from tuberculosis and our knowledge of its pathology justify this, and the improved prospect of recovery when attacked confirms this conclusion.

In Watson's *Practice of Physic* (vol. ii, p. 201) it is stated that "the tubercular disease when established is beyond our power"; and A. Ransome quotes a doggerel rhyme of the eighteenth century to the following effect

> If consumption cured can be
> Which is a mighty rarity,

These three things you must prepare,
Milk, traumatics[1] and fresh air.

A large share of the credit in reducing tuberculosis must be given to improved methods of treatment. George Bodington (1799–1882) of Sutton Coldfield, England, in his "Essay on the Treatment of Pulmonary Consumption" (1840), dwelt on the advantages of cold air in the "healing and closing of cavities and ulcers of the lungs," also of exercise in the open air and abundant nutrition. Contemporary criticism of these principles was abundant. The first consumption sanatorium was established in the Waldenburg Mountains by H. Brehmer in 1859. E. L. Trudeau soon after this began his work at Saranac, New York; and in 1876 Dettweiler began his work at Falkenstein in the Taumus. Since then the Sanatorium movement has spread throughout the world, and has had immense influence on the habits of entire communities, as well as on the patients treated in sanatoria. The love of the open air, the horror of stuffy rooms, the need for care in personal habits as to expectoration, the importance of treatment of early symptoms of illness, have all been taught and are becoming increasingly appreciated.

For the patients themselves perhaps the chief gain has been in the training given as to methods of living while they remain patients and after their discharge when improved or recovered. Many patients have

[1]Blisters or issues.

been helped on the road to health; and for very many more the risks of infection to the family of the patient or to those who work with him has been greatly reduced not only by the intermission of infection while he is in the Sanatorium, but also as the result of his more careful habits when at home. Sanatoria have been admirable colleges of hygiene.

Hospitals for consumptives during acute acerbations of illness and when the patients are permanently bed-ridden have been an important factor in diminishing the risk of infection especially when this is at its maximum. (On this see my *Prevention of Tuberculosis*, especially Chapter XXXVI.)

Reference in conclusion may be made to the argument that inasmuch as the death rate from tuberculosis was steadily declining for some years before Koch's discovery of the tubercle bacillus, and inasmuch as it did not increasingly decline after this discovery, measures against infection have counted little, as compared with indirect factors which have improved social conditions.

The argument is too simple to be credible. It assumes that factors other than infection have remained constant, and that furthermore Koch's discovery produced an immediate effect in the institution of new measures against infection; both of which assumptions are manifestly erroneous. Recent decades have been characterised by a rapid increase in the substitution of town life for country life and of indoor for outdoor occupations, factors which should have been associated with increased tuberculosis or at least a stationary death rate from this disease. But it has declined at least as rapidly and steadily in recent as in earlier decades. That action directed solely against infection from person to person can abolish tuberculosis is shown by experience with herds of cattle, from which it has been eliminated by the tuberculin test for diagnosis, and by the segregation of reacting animals; aided by the removal of the calves when born from the tuberculous cows which have borne them. Such drastic measures are impracticable for human beings; but the opportunities for infection can be greatly reduced, and indirect measures decreasing opportunities for, as well as increasing resistance to, infection are constantly available; and thus each successive crop of tuberculous infection becomes scantier than its predecessor.

# PART II

# SOME PHYSICAL AND SOCIAL CONDITIONS OF HEALTH

# CHAPTER XXI

## Air and Ventilation

Preventive medicine is concerned with the prevention of disease and with the preservation and enhancement of health. Of all the diseases from which humanity suffers, the most serious and lethal are those caused by infective agents introduced from without, and preventive medicine will continue to be largely if not chiefly concerned with them. Furthermore, to prevent infection is to adopt one of the most important measures for the maintenance and improvement of health. But such measures do not embrace the whole field of preventive medicine; and there are physical and physiological factors of health, the fundamental value of which has been revealed by the scientific developments of recent years. These might appropriately have been outlined at the beginning of this volume; but for the reason stated on page 12 and because relatively few pages can be devoted to them, they are briefly considered here.

The influence of conditions of air and ventilation, of temperature and humidity, of sunlight and, in relation especially to these, of housing conditions, and the influence of general sanitation, come within the scope of our brief review. And equally important with these is the entire subject of nutrition, of the dangers associated with unsuitable or contaminated food, and of the internal secretions of the body, the importance of which in relation to health is being slowly revealed.

In this and the following chapters an attempt is made to illustrate the above branches of hygiene, and so, it is hoped, to stimulate the reader to seek after the fuller knowledge which is obtainable from larger works.

It has long been known that air polluted with human exhalations is injurious, and such instances as that of the Black Hole of Calcutta, quoted in most text books, have given dramatic demonstration of the lethal effects of such air. In this tragedy 146 adults were confined in a room 18 feet square with two small windows. Next morning only 23 were alive.

It was supposed that this result was owing to excess of carbonic acid gas in the expired air, and this was taught by Lavoisier; but as early as 1857 Claude Bernard's experiments showed that the increase of carbonic acid gas in occupied places is far below the lethal limit.

In 1863 von Pettenkofer proclaimed the harmlessness of carbonic acid in an ordinary occupied room; but proposed to regard the amount of this gas as the index of other and more serious impurities of air. The test was useful, and is still largely employed in conjunction with criteria as to bacterial contents, dust, humidity and temperature. Dr. J. S. Haldane's $CO_2$ testing apparatus rendered possible accurate observation of $CO_2$ in air on a large scale. He disproved Pettenkofer's view that $CO_2$ is a reliable indicator of air impurities, and showed also that the reduction of oxygen does not account for the effects of bad air.

It was next assumed that "organic effluvia" in expired air were the chief enemy; and Brown Sèquard and d'Aronsal in 1887 reported that expired air contained a volatile poison. Others, however, disproved the existence of such a poison in expired air; and in 1883 Hermann pointed out that probably excessive heat and moisture are the most harmful factors in bad air, and that the discomfort caused by such air probably results from interference with the escape of heat from the body surface. In and about 1905 Heymann Paul and Erclentz made many experiments under Flügge at the Institute of Hygiene, Breslau, showing that the symptoms experienced in breathing so-called vitiated air are due to heat stagnation in the body, and that the temperature of the air, its moisture and stillness are responsible for these symptoms. Each of these elements affects the rapidity of loss of heat from the body. Thus if a person while experiencing discomfort in the experimental cabinet was allowed to breathe through a tube outside fresh air which had the same temperature and relative humidity as that within the cabinet, no relief was experienced; but immediate relief was given by a fan or by lowering the temperature of the air supplied, without any other change. J. S. Haldane and Leonard Hill have confirmed and extended these results. These results emphasize the desirability of living either in the open air, or in a room the air of which is cool and not stagnant, stimulation of the skin and heightened cell activity being increased in these circumstances.

The problem of ventilation was thus proved to be physical or thermal rather than chemical, and to be concerned more with the skin than with the lungs. In short, air is unfitted for ventilation in proportion as it loses its capacity for taking up heat.

Haldane's experiments made in 1905 showed experimentally the effect of moving as compared with still air, a relatively high temperature of the wet-bulb thermometer associated with moving air being borne without producing the higher rectal temperature, increased pulse, throbbing head, dyspnoea and general discomfort caused by the same temperature when the external air was stationary.

The Departmental Committee (Great Britain) on Factory and Workshop Ventilation, 1907, recognized the removal of excessive heat and moisture as the primary objectives in ventilation, and the New York State Commission on Ventilation (1923) after detailed experimentation found that under otherwise equivalent conditions, the output of work was reduced by 15 per cent at 75°F., as compared with 68°, and by 37 per cent at 85°F. as compared with 68°. In England similarly Vernon showed that in tin-plate works with good ventilation the summer output of work was only 3 per cent less than that in the winter months, but that without good ventilation the summer work decreased 13 per cent. An important practical conclusion from the experimental observations outlined above has been stated in the report of the New York Commission. The report of this Commission showed that the air change of 30 cubic feet per minute required by the laws in a large number of states, which had been advocated on the older physiological assumptions, was "not only needless but actually harmful to health and comfort, as it almost inevitably leads to overheating." Thus is emphasized the principle that all other factors of good ventilation of factories, lecture-rooms, etc.—such as amount of air-change and direction of flow of air—must be regarded as entirely subsidiary to the essential point, *viz.*, the avoidance of overheating of the room.

For physiological comfort and for efficiency in working, the temperature and humidity of the air respired are its most important features. Other special conditions need also to be considered. Extraneous poisonous gases are sometimes found, the most important being derived from the escape into the room of carbon monoxide, CO, derived from the combustion of illuminating and other gases. This gas is evolved in dangerous quantities in the combustion of gasoline (petrol) in an automobile in a closed garage. The replenishment of illuminating gas derived from coal by extra illuminants containing a much greater amount of CO has increased the risk of CO poisoning in recent years. Exposure to 1 part of CO in 2000 of air has proved toxic, and in half an hour exposure to 2 to 3 parts per 1000 may be dangerous to life.

But from the point of view of disease production, chief importance attaches to the dust in air. In the chapter on Industrial Hygiene, the question of dust is further considered, as also in relation to the obstruction to sunlight by fog and smoke (p. 212). Here we need only indicate a few points as to progress in our knowledge of the influence of sewer-air and drain-air on health, and our increasing knowledge as to the bacteriology of the air.

As seen in *Evolution of Preventive Medicine* "corruption of the air" was regarded as a chief cause of epidemic diseases. Thus Southwood Smith in a work on "Fever" published in 1820 said: "The immediate, or the exciting, cause of fever is a poison formed by the corruption, or the decomposition, of organic matter."

Charles Murchison in his treatise on "Continued Fevers" collected evidence which appeared to point in the same direction, and gave the name "pythogenic" to enteric fever, as embodying the same view. One instance quoted by him is that of the cleaning out of a foul privy at a school in Clapham, which was followed in 23 children by symptoms of vomiting, purging, headache, and convulsions, two of the children dying within 24 hours; apparently an instance of acute toxic poisoning. Thackrah many years earlier had, however, observed that sewer men were not specially subject to disease; but it was generally held that the air of sewers passing into houses aggravated the severity of all the exanthemata, of erysipelas, hospital gangrene, and puerperal fever. In Parkes' standard "Hygiene" 1878, page 127, the following statement appears: "That enteric fever may arise from the effluvia from sewers is a doctrine very generally admitted in this country, and is supported by strong evidence."

That this view was not universal is evidenced by the propositions laid before a meeting of the British Association in 1864, in a debate on the sewage question: (1) that atmospheric air strongly impregnated with odours of various kinds is not necessarily injurious to health; (2) that atmospheric air without smell is often most dangerous; (3) that smells, as smells, are neither injurious to health, nor are they a nuisance to those who live among them (quoted by Parkin, *Medical Times and Gazette*, October 4, 1864).

In the same discussion, Livingstone, the great traveller and apostle of Africa, while protesting against being thought "an advocate of stinks" stated that "he believed it was most important to know that stinks were not the cause of fever in Africa."

When cesspools in towns began to be abolished and discharge of the contents of water-closets and of other waste-waters into main sewers was substituted, other dangers arose, some real, others largely imaginary. The real dangers were increased possibilities of specific contamination of water-supplies, though it must be still accepted that fœtid gases getting into dwelling-rooms from leaky or blocked soil-pipes, etc., may be detrimental to health. That they were held to be much more maleficent than this indefinite statement implies was widely held. Thus in a paper on "Sewer Gas and Ear Disease," Dr. J. P. Cassells (*Glasgow Med. Chi. Soc.*, January, 1878) related a number of cases of sore throat and deafness associated with defective house-drainage, which disappeared when sanitary improvement was made.

Prince Consort, the husband of Queen Victoria, died in December, 1861 of enteric fever, supposed to have been caused by defective drainage of a house in which he had been staying. More probably it was caused, as also the nearly fatal attack of the same disease suffered a few years later by the Prince of Wales, (afterwards Edward VII) by contaminated oysters, not then recognized as a vehicle of enteric fever. In the same period the occurrence of septic complications after childbirth of one of the English royal princesses was similarly ascribed to effluvia from a defective water-closet in a room adjoining her bedroom, as can be seen by reference to a standard text-book on midwifery of that period.

The following illustrations on the same subject are taken from an admirable book published in 1883 by J. and A. Churchill, entitled *Dangers to Health* and written by T. Pridgin Teale, a distinguished Leeds surgeon.

In the first of these (fig. 8) is seen a lavatory basin untrapped and discharging into the soil-pipe leading down to the drain. This condition was found in the house of a medical man whose wife had puerperal fever, which was presumed to be due to the noxious effluvia from this pipe.

In the second diagram (fig. 9) is shown a soil-pipe perforated at several points, concealed behind boarding, which ended under the floor of the medical student's room in a broken junction with the underground drain. The student suffered from frequent sore throats. In both of these instances, the introduction of gases evolved during the decomposition of putrefying matter was probably inimical to health, though it is unlikely that these gases were responsible for the illnesses ascribed to them. In the decade 1871–1880 and even later the infection of diphtheria and enteric fever and of some other infectious diseases was generally attributed to drain effluvia, and the detection of sanitary defects allowing such emission of effluvia was regarded as an adequate investigation in causation. The importance of contaminated water, milk and other foods in this connection was but little appreciated.

Exact investigation by Carnelley and J. Haldane (*Proceedings Royal Society*, 1887) showed that in the air of the small sewers and drains of the House of Commons there was an excess of carbonic acid and of organic matter, but that there were fewer microörganisms than in outside air, from which the sewer air organisms appeared to be derived.

Nägeli in 1877 had showed that bacteria do not become detached from the liquids containing them, except by direct splashing. Even then it would be unlikely that such particulate matter would escape detention by deposition on the sides of moist pipe bends before reaching the air of rooms. Nägeli stated that "liquids or damp substances do not, with ordi-

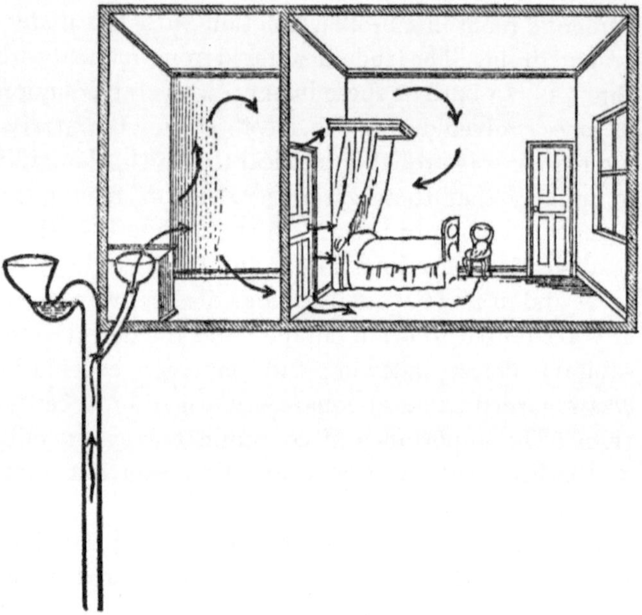

Fig. 8

nary air-currents, give off microörganisms to the surrounding air."

Similarly air drawn through gravel is deprived of any particles in it; and it will be remembered that in Pasteur's experiments (page 27) bent tubes were

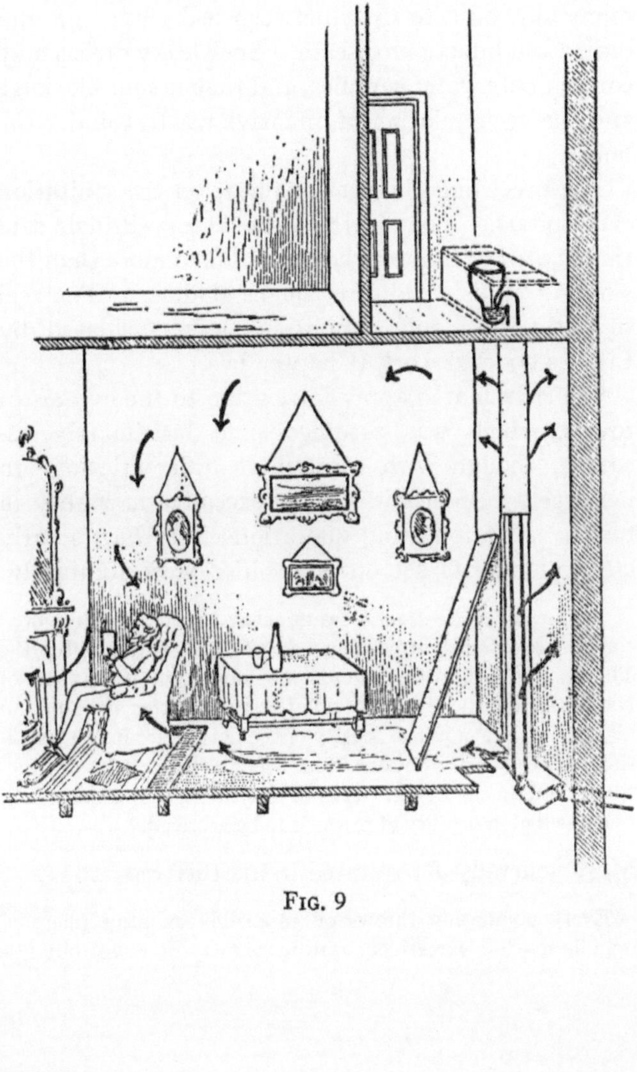

FIG. 9

used to sterilize incoming air. These laboratory observations disprove much of the association formerly supposed to exist between leaky underground drains and infectious disease. Such leaky drains may contaminate water supplies, and they favour blockage and the accumulation of offensive matters under the house.

The preceding observations bear on the sanitation of hospitals. Early in the 18th century Pringle said that the air of military hospitals killed more than the sword. "Plus occidit aer quam gladius." The real significance of such conditions was elucidated by Lister's epochal work (Chapter IV).

Similar remarks apply in relation to the evil air of towns, which was assumed—and legitimately assumed, though with incomplete differentiation—to be largely responsible for the excessive mortality in towns. The following quotations from Farr's early classical reports set out the older view admirably:

> The exhalations from sewers, churchyards, vaults, etc., commingle in this atmosphere as polluted waters enter the Thames, and notwithstanding the wonderful provisions of Nature for the speedy oxidation of organic matter in water and air, accumulate, and the density of the poison (for in the transition of decay it is a poison) is sufficient to impress its destructive action on the living. It is to this cause, it appears to me, that the high mortality of towns is to be ascribed.

More generally Farr stated in another report:

> Every population throws off insensibly an atmosphere of organic matter, excessively rare in country or town, but less

rare in dense than in open districts; and this atmosphere hangs over cities like a light cloud, slowly spreading, driven about, falling, dispersed by the winds, washed down by showers.

The influence of housing and of industrial, especially of indoor, occupations is indicated in the two next chapters; but the contents of this chapter must be completed by reference to what constitutes the chief risk of indoor air, *viz.* its *bacterial content.* Already allusion has been made to the mistaken idea that drains and sewers give off pathogenic bacteria from their wet surfaces. It may be added, in further illustration of this point, that Tyndall long ago showed that air in a closed box the walls of which had been painted with glycerine speedily lost its dust, the course of a beam of light passed through the box then becoming invisible. Nägeli in 1877 had shown that bacteria are not given off from moist surfaces; and in 1881 Tyndall showed that they are absent from expired air. (See his *Essays on the Floating Matter of the Air*, 1881.)

But this experimental evidence is compatible with the fact that the chief risk of communicating such diseases as whooping cough and measles, diphtheria and scarlet fever, and tuberculosis, is derived from the respiratory tract of the patient, not in quiet respiration, but in speaking and in coughing and expectoration. Several experimenters, including Flügge, showed that if the mouth be rinsed out with broth cultures of *Bacillus prodigiosus*, the bacilli can be caught on culture plates at considerable distances in the same room or hall, some of them being found behind the speaker, who has thus scattered bacilli in droplets of saliva while speaking. M. Gordon showed that a speaker may eject a fine spray containing bacteria for at least 40 feet from the platform of a hall. Such experiments may give an exaggerated idea of the risks of daily life; though their bearing on the transmission of a "common cold" or some of the more serious catarrhal infections is obvious. In pulmonary tuberculosis, however, exact observations show, as Cornet has put it, that "the saliva is either free from the bacilli or contains them in rare cases and in small numbers." In this disease the chief danger is incurred in intimate association with the patient, when direct infection by droplets containing tubercle bacilli is very liable to occur.

Koch as the result of experimental observations concluded that dried sputum producing dust, owing to the carelessness of patients, is a much more likely source of infection than the droplets directly discharged during coughing. He pointed out that

> The sputum is not only ejected directly on the floor, there to dry up, to be pulverised and to rise again in the form of dust, but a good deal of it dries on bed linen, articles of clothing, and especially pocket handkerchiefs. . . . and this too is subsequently scattered as dust.

(See also page 90 of my *Prevention of Tuberculosis*.)

On the other hand it has been shown that tubercle bacilli are seldom found in dust and on the surfaces of rooms, except near a patient, and then in small quantities. The details of the discrepant observations are given in the work quoted above. Here it must suffice to state that probably direct infection by droplets is the most serious risk for those in daily contact with consumptives, and that infection by dust containing dried tubercle bacilli is steadily decreasing, owing to the improved habits of patients as to disposal of sputum. The great risk, especially to children from fondling, from contact with infectious patients with unwashed hands, and from toys, spoons, etc. needs to be emphasized.

The change in perspective of teaching as to protection of wounds (page 34) may be referred to at this point. The risk from the ordinary air bacteria is relatively small, that from contact dirt is great. Many millions of bacteria are present in the floating dust of city streets. They are much more numerous than the floating bacteria in indoor air; but most of them are relatively harmless. It may be stated generally that infection by bacteria from specifically ill patients occurs chiefly, almost solely, in the immediate vicinity of these patients.

We may summarize the contents of this chapter by stating that for comfort and fitness for work movement of air and a fairly low temperature are required. These conditions also have great influence in the maintenance of good health. Sewer and drain emanations are objectionable, but they are not responsible for the dissemination of the infective material of specific febrile diseases. These are carried from patient to patient directly in droplets containing the infective material, or by actual contact on dirty fingers or eating utensils, less often in dust derived from the infective patient.

## CHAPTER XXII

### Fog, Smoke, Sunlight

More important than the extraneous gaseous contents of the air are its thermal condition and humidity (page 199), and from the point of view of disease production most important of all is the particulate matter the air may contain. The influence of smoke will be considered in this chapter, of industrial dust in Chapter XXIII.

As regards extaneous gaseous contents exception must be made of carbonic oxide (page 199) and of sulphurous acid fumes which play a large part in producing the distressing effects of foggy weather in towns.

The effect of fog and smoke in the air is due in part to its direct irritating effect, and in part to its shutting off the rays of the sun. Diogenes, asked by Alexander the Great, "can I do anything for you" made the wise answer: "Yes, get out of my sunshine." The deficiency of winter sunshine—even when this deficiency is not increased by avoidable smoke—in Britain and some other temperate countries, is their most serious climatic defect. In tropical and subtropical countries, on the other hand, continuous unobstructed sunshine, makes the clouds of the temperate zone a blessed relief, especially as,—in the absence of practicable preventive measures,—the higher temperature is followed by great excess of parasitic life.

Figures have been given showing the vast deposit of soot in towns. Thus in Pittsburgh 1031 tons, in Glasgow 820 tons and in Leeds 539 tons of soot have been deposited on a square mile in a single year. It is estimated that at least 3 times the amount of smoke emitted from industrial chimneys comes from domestic dwellings. In 1925 the annual soot fall was 35,000 tons in the whole of London, not more than half the amount of the fall some 13 years earlier (F. W. Goodenough). The Royal Commission's Report on the Coal Industry stated that "in effect the work of over a million men for three days every year is devoted to providing the soot which pollutes our atmosphere." In producing this result our domestic fireplaces are the worst offenders.

The use of soft coal as fuel began in London in the 13th century, and in Edward I's reign its use during the sessions of Parliament was prohibited.

The objections increasingly felt to smoke in towns are not only aesthetic, in the interest of cleanliness, and because it diminishes the opening of windows, but also because it shuts off sunlight, and especially the ultra-violet rays of light. According to an official statement the obstruction to sunlight results in the loss of 20 per cent of sunshine in towns of England, and probably at least 65 per cent of the possible ultra-violet rays are lost (L. Hill).

Fog adds further to the loss of light produced by

smoke, and greatly increases the retention of the irritating gaseous products of combustion. Tyndall's experiments (page 207) showed how much fine dust is contained in air, though this is only visible in bright sunlight. These particles, and still more the crowd of larger particles contained in dusty and smoky air form nuclei for condensation of water vapour, and so play an important part in promoting fog and rain. Evelyn, one of the founders of the Royal Society, referred to the "hellish and dismal cloud of sea-coal" which made the city of London "the suburbs of hell," and Russell of Glasgow some fifty years ago described with accuracy the state of many English towns in the following words:

> When in the winter we happen upon a low temperature, a high barometer and a dead calm, we have an arctic night with a mephitic atmosphere in which we move about choking, our eyes irritated, our faces grimy. . . . . It is then that our pulmonary mortality is run up, and the death rate of the year determined.

The effect of a few days of smoky fog in increasing the death rate in the following week, especially from bronchitis and other respiratory affections, is well known. Thus in two weeks in January and February, 1880, in these circumstances the total death rate in London rose from 27 to 48 per 1000 of population. How much of this effect is the direct result of the fog, and how much of the excessively low temperature associated with it, is open to doubt. W. T. Russell

(*Lancet*, August 16, 1924) after an analysis of statistics for a series of years has concluded that when fog was unaccompanied by lowering of the air temperature "no perceptible movement in the mortality curve took place." It is the combination for several days of fog, frost, deprival of sunlight and still air which is especially lethal. As a practical problem in preventive medicine, we know that removal of coal dust from the air would diminish the density and duration of the fog, reduce its irritant effect, and possibly admit a certain proportion of the sun's rays.

Our knowledge of the influence of sunlight on health has vastly increased in recent years.

In 1875 T. P. Blount and A. Downes showed that light is inimical to the development of bacteria. In 1878–1879 they proved experimentally that this result does not follow when bacteria are exposed to light *in vacuo*, but only when there is exposure to light in air. They showed also that this effect was not due to the temperature of the sun's rays.

Buchner of Munich sowed a growth of the vibrio of cholera thickly on an agar plate. Black paper letters of the word "cholera" were attached to the under surface of the plate, and the plate was then placed for 1½ hours in the sun bottom upwards. After this exposure growth of the vibrios was allowed in the dark at a suitable temperature. These grew only over the word "cholera."

At the International Medical Congress, Berlin, 1890, Koch made the following relevant statement:

As to direct sunlight, it has been well known for some years that it kills bacteria with tolerable quickness. I can affirm this as regards tubercle bacilli, which were killed in from a few minutes to some hours, according to the thickness of the layer in which they were exposed to sunlight. . . . . Even ordinary daylight, if it last long enough, produces the same effect; cultures of tubercle bacilli die in five to seven days if exposed to the window in compact masses.

The influence of sunlight in the prevention and treatment of disease will be further considered in the chapter on Rickets (page 265), but some earlier investigations may be mentioned here. In 1889 Huntley and in 1900 Palm published articles lauding sunlight as a preventive of rickets. In 1819 Raczynski (quoted by Rowland) published the first experimental evidence of the physiological effect of the sun. Puppies in the absence of sunshine assimilated less calcium and phosphorus than puppies exposed to the sun. Later experimental results are given on page 263. Mrs. Mellanby has shown that decay of the teeth is related to deficiency of sun and of food.

The separate influence of the invisible ultra-violet part of the spectrum was stated by Huldschinsky in 1919, who showed that rickets could be prevented or cured either by irradiation with sunlight or by exposure to the quartz mercury lamp. Most of these invisible rays are cut off by ordinary window glass, but not to the same extent by new kinds of quartz glass. These are partially pervious to these ravs.

Hence the importance, especially for children, of a largely out-door life, and of dress which will expose considerable surfaces of skin to the rays and to the stimulating effect on the skin and lungs of moving air.

In 1893–1894 Finsen published his work showing the value of exclusion of the ultra-violet rays of light in the treatment of small pox, and cure by their use in the treatment of lupus. The original Finsen lamps are now superseded largely by varieties of mercury vapour and tungsten arcs, while larger carbon arc lamps are usually reserved for general light baths.

In 1903 helio-therapy was used in surgical tuberculosis by Bernhard. He was followed by Rollier at Leysin and since 1908 by Gauvain and others. Gauvain has contended with force that as shown by clinical evidence, the benefits of light treatment for surgical tuberculosis are not entirely due to the ultra-violet rays of light; and Leonard Hill regards the basal metabolic changes during such treatment as due chiefly to exposure to cold air. Visible rays of light have greater penetrating power through the skin than invisible rays, and sunlight is as a rule preferable to the use of the ultra-violet rays, when the former is obtainable. The ultra-violet rays should be used under really skilled supervision.

# CHAPTER XXIII

## Housing and Occupation

Among the physiological conditions of health, air and light stand first, adequate nutrition standing on an equality with these (*primus et secundus inter pares*). Next to these comes protection against extremes of heat and cold by clothing and housing, and protection against the risks associated with one's life work.

Of housing little can be written here, notwithstanding its importance. A few salient points may, however, be mentioned. The nineteenth and the twentieth centuries have been characterized by vast improvements in the circumstances associated with home life, and by almost equally great increases in the dangers of home life. Let us look at some of these counteracting influences. Water supplies have been safeguarded. Removal of domestic refuse and especially of sewage has been organised and vast communities protected from intestinal infections. The dwelling-house has in large measure ceased to be a place for the treatment of many of the more serious diseases, treatment in hospital replacing it. The habits of the mass of the population have become more cleanly to an almost incredible extent. Modern conditions of living have rendered possible the provision by the larger family—the community—of education, recreation and locomotion, on a scale and of a quality never previously attempted.

But these and many other advantages of modern communal life have been partially counterbalanced by the risks and drawbacks associated with life in a crowd. Life in nearly all particulars has become more complicated as communities have become more urban. In every country the trend to the towns appears to be ever increasing. In England more than one-half and in the United States one-third of the total population live under urban conditions. The following figures are most impressive (Thomas Adams, *De Lamar Lectures, 1925–1926*):

*Metropolitan areas with a population of one-half million and over*

| | *Number of areas* |
|---|---|
| United States | 12 |
| Germany | 7 |
| Britain | 5 |
| France | 3 |
| China | 12 |

With this increasing urbanization has gone a more rapid growth of population; the rate of increase is now, however, abating. In 1750 England and Wales had a population of 6 millions, now of over 35 millions. The checks to growth supplied by famine, pestilence, and even war partially, have been removed; volitional restriction has largely taken their place.

The aggregation of houses in close proximity has greatly increased the risks to health. A large family with insufficient accommodation in a wilderness of houses is exposed to infinitely greater risks to physical and moral health than the same family living at the edge of green fields. R. L. Stevenson in *Prince Otto* said: "And although we should be grateful for good houses, there is, after all, no house like God's out-of-doors;" and Sir Walter Raleigh is quoted by B. W. Richardson as saying "no man has a house, unless he has a garden."

In towns there are almost universally more occupants to each dwelling room than in rural districts. Furthermore a given degree of crowding is much more serious in town than in country. For, not only is the organic filth of life more difficult to remove in towns, but the occasions on which the germs of infectious diseases, including tuberculosis, can be transmitted are multiplied a thousand fold. There is the further evil that a chief source of good conduct, the influence of public opinion,—that of one's neighbors,—is largely lost in town life, and vice, drunkenness, and injury from accident are more rife Add to these factors the momentous change from chiefly outdoor to chiefly indoor occupations, and one can then appreciate the greater complexity of modern life and the magnitude of the triumph shown by reduced disease as can be gathered in part from perusal of the chapters of this volume.

One of the great reasons for the improvement secured has been the humanising and the sanitation of industrial life, especially life in work shops and factories.

## OCCUPATIONAL HYGIENE

Practically one-third of the life of a man on an average is spent in the pursuit of his special calling in life, and during the nineteenth and twentieth centuries, the vast increase in industrial life concentrated in large centres of work has necessitated great reforms, which have slowly improved the lot of the worker. Strictly speaking, the hygiene of school work, and of the non-industrial work of women should also be reviewed, but this must be omitted, except in so far as it is included in the contents of other chapters.

In 1713 B. Ramazzini published at Padua *De Morbis Artificum*,—the first work describing some of the chief diseases associated with special occupations. In 1831 appeared the better known work by Dr. C. Turner Thackrah of Leeds, the full title of which was *The Effects of the Principal Arts, Trades, and Professions and of Civic States and Habits of Living on Health and Longevity.* From this may be quoted a comparison of the vital statistics in 1821 of a manufacturing town, a small cathedral and semi-urban city, and a rural district all in the same riding:

| | Population | Ratio of deaths to population |
|---|---|---|
| Leeds | 83,796 | 1 to 55 |
| Ripon | 12,131 | 1 to 67½ |
| Pickering Lythe | 15,232 | 1 to 74 |

Thackrah clearly recognised that the difference between these three districts was not due solely to the industrial life of Leeds; and it is still necessary to bear in mind the important distinction between social and industrial causes of disease. Thus in speaking of the excessive mortality of "gentlemen's coachmen" Thackrah refers to their having to wait for their masters, and meanwhile, to use Dr. Good's phrase, "they fill up their time by filling up their stomach."

Thackrah was equally outspoken as to intemperance. Thus on page 113:

> The grand bane of civilized life is *Intemperance.* Greater in towns than in the country, it dreadfully aggravates the evils of our employments, and it produces evils of its own, tenfold more urgent, more rapid, and more deadly.

Nor is he in doubt as to the remedy! (page 115):

> The vice of the operative reflects on the master. Much, very much, might be done to reduce this wide-spread evil. Let the master discharge from his employ every man who "breaks work;" nay, let him admonish, and afterwards discharge every man who spends his evenings in the alehouse, or calls at the dram Shop. . . . . A master can, a master ought to interfere.

An interesting light is thrown by Thackrah on a disease which now, with decreasing tuberculosis, is much less common than in the past. He quotes the instance of a tailor's shop in Pimlico, in which among the 334 men employed anal fistula was so common that they had a "fistula club."

A remarkable forecast was embodied in his words

"The employment of young children in *any* labor is wrong" (page 45).

Some of the most serious evils in industry arise from hard dust. On this point Thackrah pointed out the difference between miners in sandstone work in the north of England who suffered severely and those who worked in limestone without inconvenience. He mentioned specially the fork grinders of Sheffield who used a *dry* grindstone and died between the age of 28 and 32, while table-knife grinders who work on *wet* stones survive to the age of 40 to 50. Since then silicosis has been the subject of elaborate investigations, which have been followed by the adoption of practical preventive measures. The Miners' Phthisis Prevention Committee of South Africa, 1919, showed that the fine rock dust produced during boring caused a chronic fibrosis of the lungs, tuberculosis being superimposed on this. It is now well established that industrial tuberculosis results from protracted exposure to the dust of crystalline rock (silicosis), but not from exposure to the dust of lime and cement. It appears that a colloidal silica is formed, which acts as a tissue poison. Coal dust has even been said to be protective, and there is no excess of phthisis in miners. In the South African mines after the institution of protective measures, the death-rate among the native miners declined from 12.8 per 1000 in 1910 to 2.6 in 1919. Miner's phthisis is relatively incommunicable to a healthy person. This has been the experience both in South Africa and in Cornwall.

Phthisis is especially prevalent in certain occupations, two of which have already been mentioned. Dr. Greenhow in reports during 1859–1862 to the English Board of Health and Privy Council concluded from an analysis of the statistics of lung diseases in agricultural and manufacturing populations respectively that "in proportion as the male and female populations are respectively attracted to indoor branches of industry, in such proportion *ceteris paribus*, their respective death-rates from phthisis are increased."

This appeared to point to indoor life as almost necessarily associated with increased tuberculosis, and the records of prisoners in the Milbank Penitentiary, 1825–1842 supported this view. Dr. Baly showed that the mortality from tuberculosis in 1842 was 3 or 4 times as great among the prisoners as among persons of the same age in London generally. Stated otherwise, a sentence of 15 years imprisonment then meant a death sentence by phthisis. We now know that this association between indoor life and phthisis does not necessarily hold gold.

The subject of phthisis in relation to occupation can be further studied in the English Registrar General's Decennial Supplement for 1911–1920, as also the relative healthiness in other respects of a large number of occupations. In the following paragraphs it is only possible to give a few further illustrations of industrial mortality and of preventive measures against it.

*Phosphorus* fumes were the cause of a considerable number of cases of necrosis of the jaw, prior to the date when the use of yellow phosphorus in making matches was prohibited. This necrosis occurred in workers with carious teeth, who had been exposed to the fumes for long periods.

*Lead* is still the cause of considerable industrial poisoning, though its amount has greatly decreased, under the influence of strict regulations and official supervision. In Britain 1058 cases of industrial lead poisoning were reported to the Home Office in the year 1900; in 1923 only 337. Experiments made at Harvard University have shown that large doses of lead when ingested have less effect than small doses given experimentally by intratracheal insufflation. In house painting the removal of old paint is risky, as is also the dry rubbing down of painted surfaces, for instance, by sand paper. The dust of white lead is especially dangerous. Strict regulations are enforced in regard to lead industries. Women, for instance, owing to the miscarriages apt to occur along with other results of absorption of lead, are forbidden to take part in the dangerous processes, including house painting with lead paint.

At the International Labour Conference held in Geneva in 1921, it was unanimously decided to recommend the Governments represented to prohibit the use of white lead in paint used on the interior of buildings. The subject is one of much technical difficulty, but it may be anticipated that restrictions will ere long be adopted which will make industrial lead poisoning a rare event.

*Anthrax* is conveyed in the course of some industrial processes. "Woolsorter's disease" was first described by Spear and Bell in 1881. It occurred among wool-sorters in the district of Bradford, Yorkshire, who had to sort wool coming from Asia Minor and Persia. This wool was sometimes derived from Mohair and other sheep dead from anthrax. Acute pneumonia of a very fatal type occurred. This disease has now almost disappeared under the influence of disinfection of hides, and other precautions including exhaust arrangements which remove from the worker the dust evolved in sorting.

A considerable number of cases of anthrax have also occurred in workers in hides and skins. Butchers occasionally are infected. If inoculation through the skin occurs, malignant pustule is produced. These cases occur when anthrax has been concealed or not recognised on the farm in which it originally occurred.

During the Great War and since then a new source of malignant pustule has been recognised. A number of civilians and soldiers developed this disease on parts of the skin where a shaving brush had been used. Shaving brushes were examined and found to contain the spores of anthrax bacilli. It was subsequently ascertained that owing to war conditions the preparation of pigs' and other bristles had fallen into the hands of countries and workers who did not adopt adequate measures of disinfection, and who derived their material from countries in which anthrax prevailed. The case illustrates well the interdependence between countries in matters of health.

*Cancer* is a disease which only to a very partial extent has come within the range of preventive medicine. At the present time there is no disease on which so much investigation from many angles by a multitude of workers is being concentrated. It is recognised that early treatment of disease already begun offers the best prospect of recovery and that the importance of knowledge of symptoms of early disease and medical consultation needs to be impressed on the general public.

It is recognised also that cancer begins at points in the body which have been subjected to protracted irritation, and this again offers indications for prevention. This irritation may be non-industrial or industrial in origin. In South India cancer of the cheek is common in those who hold inside the cheek a small ball containing quicklime with other ingredients. In Cashmere the natives wear inside their loin cloth a small brazier made of clay covered with wicker work, and containing burning charcoal. It rests between the thigh and the abdomen, and is kept alive at intervals by blowing on it. Cancer at this site is common.

Chimney-sweep epithelioma on or near the scrotum was formerly common, due to friction and the chronic irritation of soot. In recent years mule-spinner's cancer has been recognised. It commonly occurs in men engaged in cotton mills between 40 and 60 years old, usually in the same position as chimney-sweep's cancer, though sometimes elsewhere. It has been traced to the soiling of parts of the body with lubricating oil with subsequent friction between the clothing and the skin. It has been suggested that friction alone is responsible for the production of this epithelioma. The conditions of prevention are obvious.

In the earlier years of work with röntgen rays, workers did not protect hands and other parts of the body exposed to the rays; and some of the workers with these rays suffered from a chronic and eventually fatal epithelioma in the exposed parts. Malignant disease of the bladder has been found to be 33 times as frequent in Bâle in workers in fuchsin and aniline factories as in the general male population.

There is some connection between alcoholism and excess of cancer. The occupational figures of the English Registrar-General show that brewers, publicans and others engaged in the manufacture and sale of alcohol suffer from excess of cancer. An investigation made by me into the statistics of groups of insured total abstainers and non-abstainers in a large insurance society showed a similar excess of deaths from cancer in the latter group. Whether the very great excess of cancer of the lips, tongue, and gullet in males as compared with females shown in English statistics is due to alcoholic habits or is largely the result of former syphilitic lesions or of smoking is not yet determined. All of these may contribute to the chronic irritation of tissues which is the usual antecedent of cancer.

## INDUSTRIAL FATIGUE

Another branch of industrial preventive medicine on which our knowledge has greatly increased is that of industrial fatigue. The earlier movement for shorter hours of work was activated by both humanitarian and hygienic motives. In 1848 Dr. W. A. Guy and others advocated in England that journeyman bakers should have at least 10 hours to themselves out of the 24; but objection was taken to legislation for this purpose, it being urged in Parliament that "it was intolerable and impossible in a free country like this to apply to labour in dwelling houses and workshops a minute system of inspection and supervision such as was found practicable in our factories." But as time passed increased restrictions on hours of labour were imposed in various industries and in particular the hours of work for children were restricted; and in this and in other respects there has been created an increased realisation that there is a human as well as a mechanical factor in industry. In the past when debate and dispute have occurred it has been assumed that the interests of production and national wealth are not the same as those of human welfare; and no effort was made on either side to test the issue experimentally, when it might be found that the two interests were after all identical.

The essential difficulty in applying this test has lain in the complexity of the human factor. The United States has led in inquiries on this subject and in promoting the application of scientific investigation to the methods and the duration of work. War experience in Britain, studied by physiologists on behalf of the Government, added much to our knowledge of the connection between hours of work and production, labour turnover, and lost time. The British Industrial Fatigue Board has issued many reports. It now works through four Committees. In addition the Naotinal Institute of Industrial Psychology directed by Dr. C. S. Myers, and similar organizations in America have done valuable work. The following figures are quoted from a paper to the Statistical Society by D. R. Wilson, the Secretary of the Industrial Fatigue Board.

Vernon tabulated the experience of a series of 29 to 90 men and of 70 to 100 women and of 17 youths engaged in munition work. The results are shown in the following table, which is self-explanatory:

| | Average hours of labour | | | Average relative hourly output | | |
|---|---|---|---|---|---|---|
| | A | B | C | A | B | C |
| Men | 58.2 | 51.0 | 50.4 | 100 | 120 | 137 |
| Women | 66.0 | 54.4 | 47.5 | 108 | 131 | 169 |
| Youths | 70.6 | 54.5 | | 105 | 127 | |

Elton (*Industrial Fatigue Research Board*, No. 6) showed that in the fine process of silk weaving productive efficiency fell about 10 per cent with even a good system of artificial light, as compared with natural lighting. Weston (Report No. 20) found a reduction in the weaving of cambric in similar circumstances. Wyatt (Report No. 22) showed that a similar but less pronounced effect occurred in the coarser processes of cotton weaving, but not always. Similar observations have shown that good weaving is handicapped when the wet bulb temperature exceeds 70° to 75°F. Psychological elements are involved in comparison of work in differing circumstances, for which allowance is difficult; but the general trend of observations like the above in rendering possible a reconcilement of the welfare of the worker with enhanced industrial efficiency cannot be mistaken.

The vast extent to which sickness and ill health interfere with industrial efficiency, and the vast possibilities of improvement, given prompt and efficient preventive and curative treatment of dental defects and errors of eyesight as well as the more common ailments of workers, may be gathered from some recent English figures given in "The Survey of Industrial Relations" of the Balfour Committee.

*Lost time in weeks*

| | 1922 | 1923 | 1924 |
|---|---|---|---|
| Sickness | 22,275,000 | 23,505,000 | 26,045,000 |
| Disputes | 3,333,000 | 1,800,000 | 1,400,000 |

Thus in 1924 the entire labour of half a million persons was lost through sickness.

# PART III

# SOME PHYSIOLOGICAL CONDITIONS OF HEALTH

## CHAPTER XXIV

### The Prevention of Goitre and Cretinism

In the metabolism which forms part of physiological life, and on the normal character of which health depends, many factors are concerned. Among these the significance of minute deficiency in the intake of some chemical substances has been demonstrated by recent discoveries as to goitre and cretinism.

The classic home of goitre is in the Alps, where also cretinism is common. Goitre may also occur in animals, and in Cleveland, Ohio, 90 per cent of the dogs have been stated to have enlarged thyroids. Rosenau states that the sheep industry in its early days was unprofitable in Michigan owing to the prevalence of goitre. In Montana there has been large loss of pigs from the same cause.

Schafer has described the thyroid secretion as "the most powerful stimulant of body metabolism known;" and when it is deficient, physical growth and mental development are both impeded. Mental dulness or even imbecility may result from its deficiency; and cretinism in the progeny is produced when there is severe shortage of it during pregnancy.

The stories of the steps which one by one led to the conclusion that goitre is a specific deficiency disease are of great interest. They demonstrate incidentally the debt of preventive medicine both to clinical medicine and to experiments on animals. The first step in our knowledge of the function of the thyroid gland was taken when Gull in 1874 associated myxœdema with thyroid atrophy in patients. But as late as 1879 Claude Bernard in his work on Operative Physiology stated we know nothing of the functions of the thyroid gland. Gull's paper (October, 1873) to the Clinical Society was entitled "On a cretinoid state supervening in adult life in women." In 1879 W. M. Ord further investigated this condition, giving it the name of myxœdema.

Theodor Kocher (1841–1917) published in 1883 an account of the effects following extirpation of the thyroid for goitre in man. This operation he had performed in some 2000 cases. He showed that in 30 of the first 100 cases of thyroidectomy a condition of "cachexia strumapriva" had followed.

Victor Horsley, experimenting on monkeys in 1885, showed that the same condition occurred in some of the monkeys whose thyroids he had removed; but these results do not appear to have suggested a remedy. But M. Schiff in papers appearing in February and August, 1884, showed that an animal could be safeguarded against some of the consequences of thyroidectomy by transplantation of a thyroid gland from another animal of the same species. He also made the remark "it would be interesting to know whether an emulsion of the thyroid gland would have an analogous effect."

In February, 1890, Horsley published a "Note

on a possible method of arresting the progress of myxœdema, cachexia strumapriva, etc.," and in 1891 Murray cured a case of myxœdema by injecting subcutaneously a glycerol extract of fresh sheep's thyroid. In 1895 Baumann discovered the normal presence in the thyroid of iodine in combination with a protein. Many years earlier the theory that iodine deficiency was responsible for endemic goitre had been advanced; and in 1905 D. Marine and others began an investigation of the relation of iodine to the glandular structure of the thyroid in man and various animals. They found that the iodine storage in the thyroid was inversely to the amount of overgrowth of the gland.

Geographically it has been found that in all races and climates, men and animals living near the sea are free from goitre; while it is endemic in certain inland districts, as in the Peak district of Derbyshire in England, in the valley of the St. Lawrence River and in the Basin of the Great Lakes (Lake Superior, etc.). It usually begins about puberty, and is more frequent in females than in males.

In 1909 Lenhart and Marine on a large scale prevented goitre in trout in a brook by adding iodine in the concentration of one part in a million.

In 1917 iodine was administered systematically to the girls attending public schools in Akron. Twice a year 2 grams of sodium iodide were administered during 14 days to 2190 pupils; of these 5 developed thyroid enlargement. Of 2305 pupils who took no prophylactic, 495 developed thyroid enlargement during the 30 months of the experiment. To 1182 pupils with goitre the same drug was given; in 773 the thyroid decreased in size. To 1049 pupils with goitre no prophylactic was given; only in 145 did the thyroid decrease.

Goitre may be regarded as the first step towards cretinism, with its characteristics of stunted physical and mental growth. This is now rapidly declining in Switzerland, under the influence of the systematized administration of minute doses of an iodine salt. Iodized table salt is now extensively used in the endemic centres of goitre in various countries. In Rochester, New York, and in some other towns the public water-supply has been iodized for the prevention of simple goitre. Some physicians have expressed fear lest the "promiscuous distribution of iodine" should prove injurious, but there is no evidence of this. There is need, however, for accurate limitation of dosage; and it appears preferable to administer the drug in suspected cases by familial rather than by municipal activity.

McGarrison in 1914 on the basis of Indian evidence has advanced the view that goitre is due to the presence in the water supply of living microörganisms. The institution of a pure water supply in a military school at Sanawar, Punjab, reduced the incidence of goitre in the children from 80 to 2 per cent, no other change having occurred. Later, McGarrison has accepted the conclusions indicated above as to the influence of iodine, while retaining his view that special microbic contamination of water or food by fœcal organisms is also involved.

Thyroxin, a crystalline substance containing 65 per cent of iodine was isolated by Kemball from the thyroid gland, and it has been produced synthetically by C. R. Harington from coal tar products and iodine; and myxœdema can be cured by a minimal dose of it.

The distribution of iodine in nature bears on the prevention of goitre. Like the fat-soluble A vitamine it is present in fair amount in milk and butter, and in large quantities in cod liver oil. It is also found in green vegetables and all dairy products; and a well-balanced and varied diet evidently is important in its prevention, as well as a diet which is free from organic contaminations.

# CHAPTER XXV

## Excesses and Deficiencies of Food

The subject of food is of perennial interest; and it has been the happy hunting ground of faddists for many years. Even now our knowledge cannot be regarded as complete. Twenty years ago the value of a dietary would have been regarded as satisfactorily stated in terms of calories; but it is now known that a diet fulfilling caloric conditions can be devised which, owing to the absence of certain accessory food factors, is incompetent to maintain life. These factors are considered in subsequent chapters, and this chapter cannot be written without some anticipation of points in Chapters XXVI to XXIX, though the intention in the following paragraphs is to consider food from a more general standpoint, in the light of historical advance of science.

There is no lack of realisation of the evil of overfeeding. Throughout the ages it has been the subject of adverse comment. Thus Thackrah in his *Diseases of Occupations* quotes a comment on the ancient Rhodians: "they built houses as if they were immortal, but they feasted as if they meant to live but a little time."

Seneca, the tutor of Nero said "many dishes make many diseases" (multos morbos, multa fercula fecerunt); and again "Count the cooks if you wonder at the mass of disease" (Innumerabiles esse morbos mirabis? Coquos numera).

Bishop Jeremy Taylor (1613–1667) similarly inveighed against the excessive eating of his day.

> Strange that for the stomach, which is scarce a span long, there should be provided so many furnaces and ovens, huge fires, and an army of cooks, cellars brimming with wine, and granaries sweating with corn; and that into one belly should enter the vintage of many nations, the spoils of distant nations, and the shell fishes of several seas.

More recently Dr. Browne Longuish writing in *The Modern Theory and Practice of Physic* (second edition, 1738) after making the wise statement that "He . . . . only deserveth the name of a good physician who always deduces his curative indications from the cause of the disease," goes on to state "Gluttony . . . . in regard to its frequency and pernicious effects ought to be placed foremost of all the antecedents of acute diseases."

Within a decade Hindhede similarly has affirmed that most disease is due to food or drink. There has (see page 278) in recent years been a great reduction in the average consumption of alcoholic drinks and an increasing appreciation of the evils of over-eating, especially for adults. The diminished consumption of meat and the increased consumption of fruit and fresh vegetables have been important factors in improving national health.

Gout is the disease which has been most definitely

associated with excessive eating and drinking. Fifty and even more so a hundred years ago, acute articular gout was regarded as a necessary evil in the life of a gentleman, and active life was interrupted at irregular intervals by this painful and disabling disease. Tophi —crystalline deposits of urate of soda—were not uncommon in the lobes of the ears of adults, associated often with similar peri-articular deposits. Now gout in its typical manifestations has become a rare disease. When most prevalent it was associated especially with the consumption of beer and of wine, especially port wine. It was seldom seen in Scotland, where whiskey was the national drink. The effects of whiskey were seen in cirrhosis of the liver, and in lesions of the nervous system.

Even now most persons aged 45 and over eat more than is desirable, and the changes associated with old age might be delayed if a more satisfactory dietary were adopted, and if adequate open air exercise were taken. These statements need modification for those engaged in laborious occupations or living in very cold climates. The Esquimau is almost completely carnivorous, apparently without the excessive blood pressure and renal disease apt to follow an excessive meat diet, though possibly only in sedentary life.

Deficient nutrition is a much more serious evil than over-nutrition; for it occurs particularly in children, in whom it prevents satisfactory growth and development, and diminishes efficiency in later life. The study of various vitamines considered in the following chapters does not cover the ground, nor can the effects of mal-nutrition be stated in terms of the production of typical diseases.

Farmers and veterinarians have recognised that cattle may be in bad condition, which is not improved until the forage supplied to them is improved in value by enriching the land on which the forage has been grown; and that prior to this replenishment cattle are especially prone to acquire infections.

There is the further fact that not all foods showing the same chemical composition have equal value. Vegetable proteins have been shown to be less digestible and less efficient biologically than animal proteins. It is becoming clear, also, that protracted dietary deficiencies which are only slight, if continued over a long period are especially injurious. Thus McCollum states: "one of the most important advances which nutrition studies have achieved in recent years is the establishment of a full appreciation of the sensitiveness of the animal body to an improperly adjusted inorganic content." This applies particularly to the calcium content of food. As an instance of a diet which is deficient in this and in other particulars may be named one which consists chiefly of white bread, butcher's meat, potatoes and sugar. To supplement, and in part to replace such a diet there is needed what McCollum has called "protective foods," especially milk and leafy edible vegetables.

It is important to note that well established disease, such as the diseases described in Chapters XXVI to

XXIX, are overshadowed in total importance by the borderline conditions which are clinically ill-marked. Our knowledge of these indefinite *dis-eases*, i.e., departures from a high standard of health, is still imperfect; but their importance is very great. It is certain that such minor imperfections in the dietary of the pregnant mother help to determine the occurrence of rickets in infants fed on an inadequate diet, which would otherwise be escaped. The same remark applies to defective dentition in young children; and there is little doubt that a considerable share in the reduction of summer diarrhoea and of respiratory affections of young children in recent years can be attributed to this improvement in maternal and infantile nutrition.

In short a satisfactory dietary must always include three foods, milk, butter and eggs; and if along with this, daily sunlight is experienced or in its absence cod liver oil is given, freedom from much avoidable illness can be ensured.

In prosperous circumstances, and even for the poor with judicious selection of food, the variety of the dietary may suffice to prevent an actual deficiency disease. But for the poor, and especially for the wives and children of wage-earning men, there is always risk that the margin of safety may, from time to time, be reached.

In children mal-nutrition may be due to other causes than an incomplete or an ill-balanced dietary. Deficient sleep, over-crowding and lack of fresh air, deficient or excessive clothing may bring about the same result, as also may septic conditions of the mouth. It may be that physical training is indicated, in aid of metabolism. Playing fields and organized games may be almost as important as better meals. Thus a given result may have a complex social causation.

The importance of this borderland of impaired health and defective development, resulting from deficient intake of certain vitamins or other food constituents has been well summarised by Hess, quoted by Cramer. Hess from his clinical experience urges clinicians to realize that

> The harmful effects of food deficiencies should not be associated in our minds essentially or chiefly with specific diseases such as scurvy or rickets, but rather as disorders of nutrition, producing slight and manifold disturbances of function. It is probable that every organ or system in the body may be affected by faulty nutrition. For example, involvement of the eyes may lead to impaired vision or nightblindness; or, on the other hand, neuritis, cardiac enlargment, disturbances of the circulating system, atrophic disorders of the skin, nails or hair, caries of the teeth, or unaccountable lack of appetite and constipation may each in turn be the earliest symptom. A more careful inquiry into the dietary of patients will result in bringing to light many cases in which vague and ill-defined symptoms can be remedied simply by rendering the diet adequate.

The special association of these food deficiences with the supply of vitamins may lead to the subject being viewed out of perspective. Cod liver oil as a preventive of rickets and extract of malt or yeast to ensure growth and development,—although admirable as supplementary measures,—are in reality makeshifts which should not be needed. The conditions of life should be such as will supply all the necessary elements of nutrition from natural foods.

Milk when boiled is deprived of some of its vitamins, but boiling or at least pasteurization is usually necessary in modern conditions of life. Skimmed milk has been deprived largely of its vitamin A (page 260). McGarrison and Osborne have shown that the prevalence of constipation is a good indicator of deficiency of vitamin A. It can be remedied by giving whole meal bread and extract of yeast.

Bread made from whole wheat is rich in vitamin B, and until roller mills were introduced some 40 years ago, this was the class of bread in use. Vitamin B was shown by Osborne and Mendel in 1919 to be almost absent from white flour. Recent work by Goldberger (quoted by W. Cramer and J. C. Mottram in *Lancet*, November 19, 1927) shows that water soluble vitamin B contains (1) a substance which is antineuritic in action and rapidly affects growth (vitamin B proper) and (2) a substance having a more delayed action on growth, and which cures or prevents a condition in animals which Goldberger regards as identical with human pellagra. These results have been confirmed by Chick and Roscoe.

The grain of wheat comprises about 2 per cent of embryo, in which is most of the vitamin B of flour.

This is mostly removed in the modern milling process; and for the very poor, who live largely on white bread this is serious. How much better would it be, were whole meal bread to become universal again, or bread made from white flour to which the germ or embryo is added in the making of the dough, than that it should continue to be necessary to supply children with extract of yeast and cod liver oil, the former of which should be entirely unnecessary and the latter only in minute quantities? It cannot be too widely known that white bread and margarine or jam make a desperately bad food for young children, while brown bread and butter is admirable, especially if an abundant supply of milk is added, and either fruit or lettuce or other green vegetables.

# CHAPTER XXVI

## Hormones and Vitamins

Chemistry and physiological experimentation have vied with each other during the last 25 years in adding to our knowledge of the functions of life and in thus extending the range of preventive medicine. Although only a few high points can be indicated in this chapter, these may serve to show how great have been the additions to our armamentarium against disease.

Urea has been made artificially. Tartaric acid has also been synthetised, including a form of this acid which acts on light like the natural acid. In the presence of ferrous hydrate formaldehyde ($CH_2O$) has been produced by the action of sunlight on carbonic acid gas in the presence of water. Furthermore formaldehyde has been synthetised by the action of ultra-violet rays on carbonic acid gas (carbon dioxide); and by this preparation of formaldehyde from inorganic matter the possible manufacture from such matter of sugar, the elements of which are arranged in multiples of the elements of formaldehyde, has been opened up.

The fixation of nitrogen from the air by electricity with formation of nitrites and nitrates has rendered possible almost unlimited fertilisation of the soil and increase of its productivity. The further discovery that formaldehyde under the influence of ultra-violet rays can be linked to nitrites to form hydroxamic acid (HO·CH·NOH), and so upward to compounds some of which are alkaloidal in nature, opens up further possibilities of increased food and nutrition.

Since Pasteur's day much light has been thrown on the part played by ferments in metabolism. Foreign proteids, i.e., proteids derived from an animal not of the same species act as a poison when injected into the veins. They do not thus act when ingested, because they are first decomposed into non-poisonous amido acids and then rebuilt up into the bodily structure. This work is effected by ferments, as is also the decomposition of ingested fat into fatty acid and glycerine, and the eventual conversion of body elements into carbon dioxide and water.

In 1902 Buchner showed that the action of living yeast cells in changing sugar into alcohol may occur when the ferment has been separated from these cells.

The discovery by Starling and Bayliss of hormones has thrown great light on many processes affecting health. This discovery is closely linked with that of organo-therapy for treatment and prevention.

In 1902 the above two observers announced the discovery of "secretin." This exists in the mucous membrane of the intestine as secretinogen, and is poured out into the intestine under the stimulus of the gastric juice. Absorbed by the veins from the intestine, it is carried to the pancreas and causes the flow of the pancreatic juice. This was the first step in the discovery of what may be regarded as chemical messengers from one organ to another. Reflex nervous impulses play an important rôle in physiological functions, but the blood carries also chemical impulses to the pancreas and other organs which determine their function. In the same way the secretion of milk may be due to a hormone received from the ovary or the foetus. Iodine metabolism is determined by the secretions of the thyroid. The functions of other endocrine glands need not be detailed here; but we are beginning to understand how greatly the adrenals and the pituitary body, for instance, affect and even determine growth and circulation, and may influence the defensive mechanism of the body against external foes. By thyroid feeding the axolotl can be converted into a terrestrial animal, its gills disappearing and lungs developing; and this is one of many instances now being discovered, which forecast future possibilities of control over human development and physiological functions. Some of the active principles determining special physiological activities have already been isolated. The momentous work of J. J. Abel and his associates in isolating adrenalin, etc., from the suprarenal gland may be cited. Thyroxin has been isolated from the thyroid gland by E. C. Kendall; and Banting, Best and Macleod have isolated the anti-diabetic hormone (insulin) from the islands of Langerhans of the pancreas. All these discoveries have opened new avenues of successful treatment of disease; and in the case of thyroid extract and thyroxin have made possible the prevention of serious disease.

Vitamins have been described by Cramer as "food hormones," and this appears to be their natural position.

Although frequent references are made to vitamins in other chapters, it is convenient to summarise here some of the chief points in the development of our knowledge of them.

The name vitamin is not entirely satisfactory. An adequate amount of protein, carbohydrates, fat and salts is also a vital necessity of health. Indeed until recent years it had been assumed by Voit, Pettenkofer, and other investigators that these four substances and water included all that was essential for normal growth and health.

In 1881, however, C. Lunin found that while mice could be maintained in good health for several months on a diet of milk alone, they always died within a month under a ration of caseinogen, milk fat, milk sugar, and the ash of milk, which comprise all the separable constituents of milk previously thought to constitute an adequate dietary. His conclusion was that other substances must be present in milk indispensable to nutrition, in addition to those enumerated above.

In 1906 Gowland Hopkins at Cambridge took two sets of rats of equal age and weight, and fed one set on mixed protein, fat, sugar and salts, and the other set on the same foods with the addition of a minimum quantity of fresh milk. The rats in the first series lost weight and became ill, those in the second series remained well and increased in weight. At the end of eighteen days the dietaries of the two groups were reversed, with a corresponding change in their physical condition. Evidently some "accessory substance" or substances were supplied by milk which were essential for health. Hopkins (*British Medical Journal*, April 26, 1919) has drawn attention to the fact that earlier observations of the adequacy of the chief foodstuffs had been made before they had been completely isolated from the foods containing them. The amount of the protective or accessory substances needing to be added for health is minute, as shown by Hopkins' experiments, but this amount is indispensable. "They must be preparations made from plant or animal tissues. They must contain something made originally by living cells. All our natural foods are parts of tissues which have lived. We ultimately owe our supply of them to the plant" (Hopkins).

In 1909 Stepp fed rats on bread and milk. They grew and multiplied normally. When the same foods had been extracted with alcohol and ether, the rats lost weight, and failed to reproduce. More recent investigations suggest the likelihood of being able to control the sexual cycle of animals by special restrictions of diet.

In 1912 Hopkins extended his observations, and gave the name of "accessory factors" to the new essentials of an adequate dietary.

In 1913 McCollum and Davies showed that an accessory factor was present in butter and eggs, but not in lard or olive oil. In 1915 they named this substance "fat-soluble A," and produced evidence of another substance, called by them "water-soluble B."

In 1913 Osborne and Mendel found that the normal growth of rats under experimentation was resumed when butter was substituted for lard.

Eijkman's researches on beri-beri published in 1897 are described on page 271. He found a definite association of this disease with feeding on polished rice. In 1911 Casimir Funk isolated a substance from rice polishings, the administration of which prevents and cures the polyneuritis in birds, produced by feeding them on polished rice. Funk introduced the term "Die Vitamine" (i.e., life amine). This particular vitamin is now known as water-soluble B. It is the anti-beri-beri or anti-neuritic factor in food.

Many workers have contributed to our rapidly increasing knowledge of vitamins, and the number of probable vitamins is probably considerably more than the four which are generally recognised.

Vitamins A and D have only been imperfectly differentiated. They represent constituents which are responsible respectively for normal growth and for the prevention of rickets. Some of the confusion between the two has been owing to the non-standardisation of the synthetic diets used in animal experimentation by different workers. Keratomalacia in children appears to arise when there is a greater deficiency of A and D than that which suffices to stop growth and produce rickets. Green vegetables contain a rich supply of vitamin A, but relatively little vitamin D. Experiments made by Luce in 1924, and by Chick and Roscoe in 1926 showed that a ration rich in green fodder increased vitamin A in milk, but only slightly influenced the anti-rachitic factor. The practical difficulty is to produce enough vitamin D in winter milk.

It has recently been found that the liver fats of cattle and sheep yield many times as much of vitamins A and D as an equal quantity of cod liver oil. This implies that there is available for children a food of great value which is free from the unpleasant flavour of cod liver oil. (See also page 256.)

Protection against both rickets and keratomalacia, and against the perhaps almost equally important antecedent conditions of these clinical entities, is given by a diet which contains whole milk, butter fat, the yolk of eggs, or the green leaves of edible plants. No protection is afforded by oils of vegetable origin. In childhood milk is the main source of protection, hence the importance of its quality, including the dairy and farm conditions in which it is produced. The protection can be rendered complete by the addition of a small amount of cod liver oil to the daily dietary of the expectant mother and of the infant after birth. McCollum has shown that cod liver oil can be heated to an extent which destroys its power to cure keratomalacia, while leaving its restraining power over the production of rickets untouched.

Mrs. Mellanby's experiments showed that puppies fed on cod liver oil along with laboratory food had perfect and regularly spaced teeth; butter was a somewhat less efficient substitute. The dentures of dogs to whom linseed oil was given instead of butter or cod liver oil were very imperfect. Dr. Mellanby has shown that an excess of cereal food, for instance, oatmeal, favours rickets, an experimental observation which bears on what is said on page 261 as to the need for a balanced diet.

The anti-beri-beri vitamin (vitamin B) is present in whole meal flour, in whole barley, in oatmeal, in unpolished rice, rye, nuts, milk, eggs and liver, etc. It is absent from canned meats, from sago, tapioca, white flour, etc. Beri-beri prevalence in certain countries is largely due to the introduction of modern milling machinery which removes the aleurone layer of rice along with the pericarp. It works similar mischief in the grinding of wheat. As Hopkins has suggested beri-beri would probably be as widely prevalent in Western countries as in the East, if decorticated wheat deprived of its germ were a sole food to the same extent as rice is in the East.

The hypothetical anti-scorbutic vitamin C is present in oranges, tomatoes, and many other fruits and in green vegetables. Milk has slight anti-scorbutic power, its amount depending on the fodder of the cow. Dried milk does not entirely lose its anti-scorbutic power, though there should be a supplementary allowance of some anti-scorbutic in the infantile diet (page 269).

McCollum and others have observed that guinea pigs suffer from scurvy even when fed on oats and all the fresh milk they will consume, although milk is a complete food. They found that these animals suffered from constipation, and that when an aperient was given regularly no scurvy arose. They then prepared an artificial orange juice containing every known constituent of the orange, and found that this was protective when added to the diet of oats and milk. These experiments appeared to suggest that scurvy may be due to toxic infection of the cæcum. Such a condition would doubtless aggravate the tendency to scurvy, but both experimental and clinical observation point to the specific influence of an anti-scorbutic substance in certain foods.

The effect of cooking on vitamins has been made the subject of investigation. It has already been noted that the amount of each of them which is essential for life is minute; but they are all easily destroyed by heating in the presence of air. A normal adult diet comprising fresh milk and meat and fresh vegetable foods ensures an adequate supply of vitamins, unless it is destroyed by excessive cooking. Vitamin A in butter, Hopkins showed, was destroyed by heating the butter to 120°C. for 4 hours if oxygen was made to bubble through the butter; but this did not occur when the butter was heated without aeration.

Milk heated to 145°F. (63°C.) for 30 minutes loses more of its anti-scorbutic potency (vitamin C) than milk kept for a few minutes at a temperature of 212°F., illustrating the fact that duration of heating in the presence of air is even more detrimental than exposure to a much higher temperature for a short time. Vitamin B is more resistant to heat than vitamin C. Prolonged stewing probably destroys all of the vitamin C which may be in the materials of the stew, and most of vitamins A and B. The vitamins in milk are unstable; and pasteurization destroys the vitamin C, and some of the vitamin A in it. Vitamins slowly oxidize on keeping, but vitamins A and D are stable in cod liver oil kept for a considerable time, only stable for some months in tissued meat. Vitamin B can be preserved in the dry state as in unpolished rice or whole meal flour.

The acids in lemon juice help to preserve the large amount of vitamin C which it contains. Dried lemon juice retains its vitamin C longer than a liquid preparation. Tinned tomatoes are stated by Hess to retain their vitamin C with little loss for three years. Germinating peas give an abundant supply of vitamins in circumstances in which it is otherwise unobtainable. Cod liver oil contains more than 200 times as much vitamin A as butter, and yeast is the richest source of vitamin B. Germinating seeds contain much of vitamins B and C and green vegetables and tomatoes contain large quantities of vitamins A, B, C and D.

The above statements although approximately correct evidently represent a transitional stage of science. Our knowledge will become more exact as time progresses; and this progress will almost certainly demonstrate the superiority of natural foods over artificial products—often sold at extravagant prices—intended to supplement deficiencies in our daily food.

Very recent investigations of Drs. Green and Mellanby have shown that animals fed on a diet deficient in vitamin A die with some infective or pyogenic lesion. They suggest that vitamin A should no longer be known as the "growth-producing vitamin," but as the "anti-infective vitamin," and that special articles of diet, such as liver, may in winter be a partial shield against bronchitis, pneumonia, and other seasonal diseases.

# CHAPTER XXVII

## The Prevention of Rickets

Rickets is a disease of early childhood, characterised by various bony deformities, due to deficient calcification of the bones. Among these a pigeon-breasted condition occurs, which limits respiration, and increases the risk of death if the child suffers from bronchitis or pneumonia. For the same reason attacks of measles and whooping cough are much more frequently fatal in rickety than in normal children. A bow-legged condition usually owes its origin to rickets; and rickets in childhood means reduced stature when adult life is reached. More serious than the deformities of limbs is the deformity and constriction of the pelvis which occurs in female rickety children. In women this becomes the most common cause of difficult, protracted, and complicated parturition: thus infantile rickets is an important cause—twenty or more years later—of mortality of mothers in childbirth, which is entirely avoidable.

Rickets affects children between the ages of two months and two years. It has been a very common disease of childhood in England and in other countries. In some towns more than half the children are said to suffer at some time and in some degree from rickets; and this proportion is probably reached if the cases are included in which the disease does not proceed so far as to produce actual bony deformities. Some data as to bony deformities resulting from rickets, given by Dr. H. P. Newsholme, and derived from an investigation of school children in the North Riding of Yorkshire may be adduced. Out of 262 known cripples under the age of 16, 14 per cent were crippled in consequence of rickets in childhood. Among nearly 13,000 school children examined 3.9 per cent of the boys and 1.7 per cent of the girls showed some degree of deformity due to past rickets. When only serious conditions were reckoned such as knock-knee, bow-leg, pigeon-breast and deformed spine which are of material concern to the future prospects of the child, one boy in every 50 and one girl in every 100 showed a marked bony deformity due to rickets.

The rickety children were shorter and lighter than the average for their age, and this poorer physique continued throughout the whole of school life in the elementary school. An important additional fact was discovered in the children showing deformities from past rickets. They were definitely backward in their education and continued so throughout school life, when compared with the average attainment of all the children under the same general conditions of environment. In this investigation there was no obvious excess of rickety deformities in the towns as compared with rural areas.

The first monograph on rickets was by Glisson (1650). Rickets had appeared in the London Bills of Mortality 17 years earlier. It is doubtful if it is altogether a modern disease, although ancient sculptures are said to give no evidence of rachitic deformities. Rickets occurs in all latitudes from Italy to the north of Scotland, and in both hemispheres. It has a seasonal incidence, being most frequent in winter and spring.

The value of cod liver oil in the treatment of rickets has long been known. Trousseau appears to have learned its value from Bretonneau. In recent years great additional light has been thrown on the causation and prevention of rickets; and its prevalence is now rapidly decreasing. Many workers—among whom Mellanby and McCollum, Osborne and Mendel, Hess and Findlay may be specially mentioned,—have contributed to this enlightenment. Other names are mentioned in the paragraphs dealing with the influence of sunlight.

Two chief views of the causation of rickets are entertained; but as our knowledge extends further, complexities of causation emerge. According to one view it is a "deficiency disease" due to defective supply—either to the mother or to the affected infant —of certain constituents of food: or it is a product of indoor life, of defective air, sunlight, and exercise.

Experiments on rats and puppies have been adduced in favour of these discrepant generalizations. Perhaps the different animals employed in the experiments may account in part for the dissimilarity of experimental experience. E. Mellanby first showed that rickets can regularly be produced in animals by a diet consisting of a minimum amount of skimmed milk, unlimited bread, with salt, orange juice and yeast. When cod liver oil was added to this diet no rickets developed in the experimental animals. Vegetable oils had no anti-rachitic effect. It was also found that heating the cod liver oil to 120°C. for four hours did not deprive it of its anti-rachitic properties (page 252). Substances preventing rickets are rich in fat-soluble A vitamin (page 251), and in the vitamin D associated with it in foods.

Findlay and Noel Paton repeated Mellanby's feeding experiments on animals kept in the country, and found that—unlike laboratory animals—these did not develop rickets on the defective diet. On the other hand Mellanby confined animals in a laboratory on a good diet and secured the absence of rickets. He also demonstrated the remarkable curative effect of cod liver oil on rachitic animals, justifying the clinical experience that this oil is a specific remedy of the first rank.

Radiographic evidence showed that deposition of calcium salts occurred in the bones within two or three weeks after the beginning of treatment by cod liver oil.

Experimental evidence and direct observation on children have demonstrated that air, sun, and exercise as well as the reception of an adequate amount of protective food are important in the prevention and cure of rickets; but experimental evidence and its balanced consideration favour decidedly the conclusion that the essential need in prevention and cure is the reception of adequate vitamins A and D, or rather of the foods in which they are most wholesomely supplied. But it cannot be said that the pathogenesis of rickets has yet been completely elucidated, though enough is known to enable it to be entirely prevented.

Scurvy also is a deficiency disease (vitamin C) and so is beri-beri (vitamin B). In these diseases the deficiency is relatively simple, and is solely responsible for the disease: in rickets there is involved the question of balance of diet, as well as of deficiency of a special vitamin.

McCollum and his co-workers have produced rickets by disturbing the quantitative relation of calcium and phosphorus in the diet; and McCollum (*Congress of American Physicians and Surgeons*, vol. xii, 1922) defines rickets as "due to an unfavourable relation between the content of calcium, of phosphate, and of a substance which is common in cod liver oil, and which occurs in various foods. It involves therefore three dietary factors in its etiology." The conception of the importance of "balance and inter-action of dietetic elements" is emphasised by Mellanby, who has shown experimentally that an excess of cereal food, like oatmeal, may lead to an increase of rickets in animals. The excess of cereal foods may imply a reduction of milk and other more important children's foods to a dangerous extent, or a disproportion between the different foods; and Mellanby lays stress on "the new conception that the various essential elements of the diet are so inter-dependent that many dietetic problems must be considered from the point of view of balance, and it is no longer possible to speak of causes or deficiencies of substances in an absolute way."

Most articles of food are poor in calcium; milk is especially rich in calcium, and contains calcium and phosphates in the right proportion. Bread is poor in calcium but has a large excess of phosphates. The important conception of a balanced diet naturally arises out of the fact that rickets is a phenomenon of growth. It only occurs in young animals, in whom unbalanced food and special dietetic deficiencies are supremely dangerous.

Milk supplies adequately both the mineral salts and the anti-rachitic vitamin needed to avoid rickets and to promote growth; and it may even be said that a shortage of milk or of its equivalent values,—whether for the mother during pregnancy, or for the infant in the first two years after birth,—is in practical life responsible for the rickets in the community.

The story of the source of the anti-rachitic power of milk and other foods has great importance. The anti-rachitic contents of foods are developed under the influence of sunlight. These elements are not, so far as we know, produced in the animal body, though they may be stored in it. Animals in the end derive their vitamins from green vegetable foods.

Thus as regards cod liver oil: the cod feeds on smaller fish, and these on the abundant spring growth of algae and microscopic green plants in the Northern seas. The vitamins derived from these become concentrated in the cod's liver. This view may need to be modified in view of recent investigations on ergo-sterol derived from cholesterol (page 264), and of what is written below.

The vitamins A and D in cow's milk are similarly derived from their green food. The milk of stall-fed cows contains but a scanty amount of vitamins: this amount can be greatly increased by giving the cow cod liver oil with its food. Cod liver oil, the yolk of egg, and beef suet all have anti-rachitic power; but vegetable oils such as olive and cotton seed and linseed oils do not possess it. Lard has it only slightly.

Recently it has been found that foods may be irradiated and thus rendered potent to prevent rickets. Milk, for instance, can be treated with the emanations from ultra-violet rays from a quartz-lamp, and its anti-rachitic efficiency thus obtained has been demonstrated both on experimental animals and on infants. It has recently been found, also, that vitamin D is produced by the action of ultra-violet rays on ergosterol, apart from living tissues.

There is thus opened out a wide possibility of irradiation of winter foods, the development of which will be very important for town dwellers.

Rosenheim and Webster have given strong reason for concluding that the irradiation of ergo-sterol is the factor in the cure of rickets. This substance was at first thought to be cholesterol, a substance present in all animal living cells. The ergo-sterol is contained in cholesterol in minute quantities; and experimentally it has been found to be the most potent means of preventing rats fed on a ricket-producing food from developing the disease.

Ergo-sterol was first isolated from ergot. It is contained in yeast and in other foods. L. Hill states that $\frac{1}{20,000}$ mgm. of ergo-sterol given to rats fed on a defective dietary will prevent the development of rickets. Ergo-sterol is now becoming available as a possible substitute for cod liver oil. If the claims for this substance are substantiated, its administration will probably be a very economical substitute for the provision and daily giving of quartz-lamp baths for the prevention and cure of rickets.

It has already been stated that rickets is a winter disease. It attains its maximum prevalence at the end of March. Evidently then climate and especially sunlight have a marked influence on its prevalence. This was demonstrated during the three years 1919–1922 by Dr. Harriette Chick of the Lister Institute and others working in Pirquet's clinic in Vienna. At that time nearly all children in central Europe were more or less rachitic. The children in the above clinics were receiving a diet which was poor in anti-rachitic substances. In all alike rickets could be prevented or cured by the addition of cod liver oil to the unsatisfactory diet. It was further proved that even an unsatisfactory diet failed to produce rickets if the children thus fed had adequate exposure to sunlight or artificial sunlight.

These results confirm what had already been determined by animal experimentation. Huldschinsky's experiments in 1919 showed the way. He was able to treat rickets successfully by radiation from a mercury vapor quartz lamp. Then Hess and Unger showed that sunlight alone was effective without the aid of emanations from an artificial source. Experiments on rats have demonstrated that when these are fed on a diet which produces rickets, this result can be prevented by daily exposure of the rats to sunlight. It might be assumed that the anti-rachitic vitamin in these circumstances is manufactured (as in the production of this vitamin in irradiated milk) in the tissues of the animal, and this view cannot be excluded at present. In all probability, however, the sunlight, whether natural or artificial does not supply additional anti-rachitic vitamin but favors prevention of rickets or recovery from it by aiding and increasing the absorption of the deficient protective materials from their scanty contents in food. Cramer and Drew have shown also that light acts as a stimulus to the production of blood platelets, and thus strengthens the defensive mechanisms against bacterial invasion from the intestine (W. Cramer, *Lancet*, May 26, 1923). But whatever the exact mechanism it is the fact that in young children rickets can be prevented by daily exposure to sunshine, or by exposure for two to five minutes daily to the emanations from a mercury vapor lamp placed at a distance of two feet.

Ordinary window glass filters out the rays which give protection against rickets. These rays are stated by A. F. Hess to be in the ultra violet zone, about 300$\mu$ in length or shorter. Special window glass is now available, which allows a portion of these rays to pass through it.

The two following statements appear to me admirably to sum up the contents of this chapter.

Cod liver oil, as expressed by H. J. Gerstenberger is "civilization's excellent, economical and practical substitute—at least during the colder and darker half of the year—for exposure to sunlight." Even if it be replaced by ergo-sterol, it will be necessary to bear in mind that vitamins derived from natural foods are always more valuable than vitamins artificially extracted. From this point of view Park's statement (*Dental Cosmos*, February, 1923) gives a balanced judgment, which may be entirely endorsed.

I believe that if pregnant women received ample well-balanced diets, in which green vegetables were abundantly supplied and cows' milk was regularly taken, and they were kept a sufficient part of their time in the open air and sun, and their infants were placed in the direct rays of the sun for a part of each day and were fed on cod liver oil for the first two or three years of life, more could be accomplished in regard to the eradication of caries of the teeth than in all other ways put together and that rickets would be abolished from the earth.

# CHAPTER XXVIII

## THE PREVENTION OF SCURVY, BERI-BERI AND XEROPHTHALMIA

Scurvy, like goitre and rickets, being a "deficiency disease," should be considered here. The earlier history of its prevalence and prevention has been outlined in my *Evolution of Preventive Medicine*, Chapter XXI, and what follows is supplementary to that chapter. The social circumstances which led to its abolition from the Navy and the Mercantile Marine were (1) the compulsory administration of a daily dose of lemon juice; and (2) the introduction of steam power and other improvements rendering voyages shorter and the provision of fresh meat, fruit and vegetables practicable. It is illustrative of the slow progress of accurate knowledge, that although Lind's work on scurvy was published in 1754 his advice as to the treatment and prevention of scurvy was ignored until 1794 when the compulsory daily naval ration was initiated and, a further interval of equal length elapsed before the same compulsion was enforced for the Mercantile Marine.

So far as sailors in London Port are concerned the following figures of admissions of cases of scurvy into the Dreadnought and Seamen's Hospital from 1852–1889 (given by Dr. Curnow in the *Lancet*, August 15, 1891) are of interest:

| | *Yearly average number of cases* |
|---|---|
| 1852–67 | 88.6 |
| 1869–75 | 22.1 |
| 1876–82 | 30.7 |
| 1883–89 | 8.3 |

Some experiences have been quoted as throwing doubt on the specific influence of lemon juice in preventing scurvy. Thus in 1850–1854 Arctic relief ships were sent to search for Sir John Franklin, and his associates. These relief ships were supplied with lemon juice of good quality, and no scurvy occurred notwithstanding great privations. But in two ships *Alert* and *Discovery* commissioned by Captain Nares for an attempt to reach the North Pole, and with superior equipment in all respects to the above, serious scurvy occurred in their first winter. A commission of inquiry failed to discover the reason for this; but on page 104 of volume II of the *Medical History of the Great War* is given a probable explanation. This states that no cognizance had been taken of the fact that the "lime juice" provided in 1875 was the preserved juice of West Indian limes, whereas in the 50's juice of Mediterranean lemons had been supplied.

The suggestion that tainted food is primarily concerned in the production of scurvy is not sustained.

The experimental study of scurvy began with the discovery of Holst and Fröhlich in 1907–1912 that the disease is produced in guinea pigs regularly when they are fed solely on a diet of oats or bread and bran and water. Holst and Fröhlich in 1912 produced scurvy in guinea pigs by a diet of cereal grains, and in 1895–1896 Theobald Smith had made a similar observation (Rosenau). The distribution of the anti-scorbutic factor in nature has been demonstrated by Miss Chick and other workers of the Lister Institute. Lind knew that dried vegetables lose their anti-scorbutic properties, and yet this important knowledge has been repeatedly ignored. Fresh vegetables and the potato stand out prominently as anti-scorbutic. It has been shown experimentally, that fresh lemon juice is four times as effective as fresh lime juice. Cooking has a detrimental effect; boiling is less harmful than prolonged cooking at a lower temperature. Jam and tinned and bottled vegetables and fruits usually lose their anti-scorbutic value. Boiled potatoes in this respect are superior to potatoes recooked or fried. The tomato is rich as an anti-scorbutic. Fürst has shown that cereals and pulses,—which possess no anti-scorbutic property,—acquire it by germination: and this knowledge proved of great value in Mesopotamia during the Great War. This applies also to germinated barley before it is kilned. Antiscorbutic liquids retain their property longer in acid solution. Fresh meat, contains but little of the anti-scorbutic vitamin C.

Unheated cows' milk as a rule contains enough vitamin C for an infant, but there is less of it in cows fed on oil cake and hay during the winter months.

Barlow's disease or scurvy in children, like adult

scurvy is characterised by pallor, and weakness and tenderness of limbs. The gums become spongy and haemorrhagic swellings occur in the limbs. This disease was described by Barlow in 1889; and he gave explicit directions as to its treatment by orange juice, potato, raw milk, and raw meat juice. As early as 1878 Cheadle had given similar directions as to infant's food generally.

J. F. Still (*Journal of Royal Society of Medicine*, January, 1925) has urged the use of "potato cream" in the treatment of scurvy, the potato flour being obtained from a potato baked in its skin. As a prophylactic he recommends orange juice rather than potato, as less likely to produce dyspepsia.

Breast-feeding is the best prophylactic against infantile scurvy, though if the mother's dietary is unsatisfactory, this may fail. The anti-scorbutic properties of cows' milk are not lost by heating it rapidly until it just reaches boiling point, and then cooling it quickly. Dried milk does not completely lose its anti-scorbutic power; but infants fed on it should have in addition small quantities of orange or tomato juice. The various patent foods containing dried milk and malted cereals are serious producers of scurvy. Most "patent" foods are to be avoided, even when they are advertised as containing vitamins.

## BERI-BERI

The way in which beri-beri was eliminated from the Japanese Navy has been told in *Evolution of Pre-*

*ventive Medicine* (page 198). This disease is characterised by weakness and loss of appetite followed by dropsy and by tingling and weakness of the legs, and more or less complete anæsthesia.

The disease is endemic in rice-growing communities in the East, where the diet is almost exclusively confined to this single cereal. At first it was thought to be due to contaminated or partially decomposed rice, just as pellagra has been ascribed to maize in a similar state. Its true pathology has now been completely elucidated by animal experimentation.

Eijkman in 1897 showed that in fowls, neuritis, with degeneration of peripheral nerves, is produced by feeding them with white or polished rice. The disease is fatal if the diet is persisted in, but the symptoms disappear if native rice is substituted in which the husk has been removed by steaming or by hot water. It may be noted that the rice grain consists of a pericarp or husk, a thin aleurone layer below this, and then the main substance containing the endosperm. The protective substance against beri-beri (vitamin B) is contained in the aleurone or "silver skin." Sir Gowland Hopkins (*British Medical Journal*, April 26, 1921) quotes the human observations made by the Dutch physician Eijkman on 279,621 persons who were prisoners in Dutch East Indies in 1897:

In 37 prisons unpolished rice was supplied: In only 1 prison, cases of beri-beri occurred.

In 13 prisons polished mixed with unpolished rice was used: In 6 prisons cases of beri-beri occurred.

In 51 prisons only polished rice was used: In 36 prisons cases of beri-beri occurred.

Reckoned per 10,000 prisoners: (a) with unpolished rice, 1 case; (b) with polished and unpolished rice, 416 cases; (c) with polished rice, 3900 cases.

Fraser and Stanton, 1909–1911 made a further demonstration in the Federated Malay States. Among 300 Japanese laborers in the virgin jungle, a division into two equal parties was made, the first having polished rice as their staple food, and the second under-milled rice retaining its pericarp. In three months beri-beri appeared in the first group, not in the second. Then polished rice was discontinued, and no further cases occurred. Later the diet of the two groups was reversed with a consistent sequence of illness.

Rosenau describes a similar experiment made in the Philppines by Strong and Cowell at a later date.

In 1911 Funk isolated a substance from rice polishings (vitamin B) which prevents and cures phyneuritis in birds (see page 251). In January, 1916, there was beri-beri among the British troops in the Gallipoli peninsula (Lieutenant Colonel Willcox, vol. ii, *Medical History of the War*). Up to February, 1916, there had occurred 342 cases of beri-beri in the troops in Mesopotamia, yeast preparations, such as marmite, being very successful in preventing and curing it. Willcox found also that bread made with

25 per cent of atta, a coarsely milled flour which is rich in anti-beri-beri vitamin, was an important help in reducing beri-beri among the troops. (See also page 253).

## KERATOMALACIA (XEROPHTHALMIA)

This although a relatively rare disease is important in the history of dietetic preventive medicine. In Europe it has occurred, curiously with exceptional frequency in Denmark, which produces butter and dairy produce in very large quantities. These are important sources of vitamin A, the protective substance against this disease; but as Denmark exports these products largely and during the Great War exported an exceptionally large proportion of its total produce, and substituted margarine for butter, evil consequences followed. In these circumstances sore eyes occurred with inflammation of the cornea, going on if unchecked to perforation of the cornea and complete blindness. These cases were investigated by Dr. C. E. Block of Copenhagen (on "Xerophthalmia" and "Dystrophy in Infants and Young Children" (*Journal of Hygiene*, January, 1921).

In certain state institutions for children 40 cases of this disease occurred in the five years 1912–1916 and 23 cases in the single year 1917. During 1918 a sudden change occurred, there being only one slight case; and no cases occurred subsequently. This improvement coincided with the addition of butter as part of the dietary of all and the preliminary administration of cod liver oil. The detailed investigation showed that the prevalence of the eye condition during the period of deprivation of butter was in proportion to the amount of whole milk which had been consumed in different groups of children.

In an industrial school in Britain, a similar outbreak occurred in 1919 and was investigated by Findlay. He found that the food supplied to the boys had been cooked in screwed down metal containers, this destroying its vitamin A. The disease disappeared when cod liver oil and swede juice were added to the dietary.

Experiments on animals have shown that when they are fed on diets lacking vitamin A conjunctivitis and corneal mischief develop similarly.

In view of the above results it is probable that a deficiency of this vitamin may be sometimes responsible for a lowered resistance to pulmonary and other infections (see page 241).

## PELLAGRA

Pellagra is a disease characterised by skin eruptions and various digestive disorders; also by nervous irritability, tremors, mental disturbances and even convulsions. It is probably due to dietetic deficiency, though there is still doubt as to its exact genesis. It has long been regarded as a food intoxication due to the toxic products of spoiled maize. It has also been attributed to auto-intoxication, or to some unknown infective agent.

It has a limited geographical distribution in Southern Europe, the Balkans, Lower Egypt, Mexico, the West Indies and the United States, but sporadic cases occur elsewhere. It occurs chiefly in maize-growing countries.

In the States many thousands of cases have been reported, with a case-mortality as high as 40 per cent. In the Southern States over a hundred thousand cases have been reported in a single year.

Dr. J. Goldberger has shown that in the States pellagra develops when the dietary is persistently poor in animal protein; and it would appear that the protein of seeds, as of wheat and maize, fails to supply all the physiological needs of mankind. Pellagra is common in the Southern States in which the commonest food consists of cereals and fat pork; it is only sporadic in the Northern States in which there is a more mixed dietary. It may occur in persons apparently well-nourished, and in them is associated with an increase of intestinal putrefaction (C. Voegtlin, *Harvey Lectures*, New York, 1919–1920). Experience in the treatment of patients in hospitals has proved that the pellagra fails to improve if the preceding defective diet is continued; but rapid improvement is secured if milk, egg and meat are added. In France pellagra disappeared with an improved dietary.

There is a definite inverse relation between local or national prosperity and the occurrence of pellagra; and it may even be said that prosperity is the chief means of prophylaxis against this disease. This, however, obviously is an unsatisfactory and incomplete analysis of its causation. It contains an important complex truth, comparable to the omnibus statements that filth produces intestinal diseases or that marshes breed malaria. Happily in these instances a nearer approach to accurate causation can be made; and for pellagra it can be said that even assuming persistence of poverty, the disease can be obviated by an adjustment of the expenditure on food which is within the reach of nearly all.

# CHAPTER XXIX

## Prevention of the Alcoholic Evil

In the study of the history of food and drink in relation to health that of the use and abuse of alcoholic drinks is perhaps the most important problem. Alcoholic drinks in the past have been drunk by a large section of most communities, and have proved to be one of the greatest foes of health and long life. The politics of restriction of alcoholic drinking fall without the scope of this chapter; but the economics of alcoholic consumption, as affecting health, and some statement of the personal and social evils wrought by them on the individual and on the community, cannot be omitted from discussion, especially in view of the fact that indulgence in alcohol has serious bearings on child hygiene and on family welfare, on the occurrence of accidents and crime, and on the liability to tuberculosis and insanity, and to exposure to venereal infection.

In the widest extent of the United States the amount of alcohol now consumed, medicinally, for sacramental purposes, and as the result of home brewing and fermentation and of illegal importation, is very much less than was consumed in past years. It is limited to certain sections of the population, or to occasional surreptitious indulgence of a somewhat larger part of the community. For these, as all are aware, there has arisen the new danger of sophisticated drinks, containing large or small amounts of wood alcohol. This may and often does cause blindness and convulsions and may be lethal in its effect.

That in the United States the evil of alcoholic drinks has been extremely serious in the past is well known. It is only necessary to quote in authoritative confirmation of this statement the following extract from a judgment of the Federal Supreme Court of Judicature which was given November 10, 1890:

> The statistics of every state show a greater amount of crime and misery attributable to the use of ardent spirits obtained at these liquor shops than to any other source. . . . .
>
> By the general concurrence of opinion of every civilised and Christian community, there are few sources of crime and misery to society equal to the dram shop, where intoxicating liquors in small quantities to be drunk at the time, are sold indiscriminately to all persons applying.

In Great Britain there is abundant evidence of continuing social mischief caused by alcoholic excess, although the average amount of alcohol consumed per capita has greatly declined. The story of the measures which have led to this gradual improvement and a general discussion of the problems involved, including the general problem of compulsory restriction, will be found in Chapters X, XI, XVI, and XVII of my *Health Problems in Organized Society* (P. S. King, 1927). Here we are only concerned with a statement of the personal and communal effects of this indulgence.

Something like one-fifth of the entire earnings of the wage-earners in Britain is still spent in alcoholic drinks, and this expenditure—an average statement implying a much higher expenditure in thousands of families—signifies that in these families women and children are deprived of necessaries of life and of the possibility of adequate nutrition and growth.

The injurious effects of alcohol may be considered as they affect the family and the community and in relation to personal welfare. In the latter connection it is necessary to distinguish between what experience and scientific experiments have proved as to the effect of small and large doses respectively.

The influence of inebriety—which may stop far short of drunkenness—in producing crime is shown in all statistical returns. The Home Secretary of England (the member of the Government responsible for judicial and police control in the country) stated in 1925 that "during the years 1923 and 1924 one-fifth of the men who went to prison, and one-half of the women, went for drunkenness. . . . ." "It would reduce enormously the prison population and the cost of maintenance if they could get rid of the crime of drunkenness altogether."

In the address from which the above remarks are quoted the Home Secretary added that "the Medical Officer of Pentonville Prison (a large metropolitan prison) had examined the cases of 40,000 men, and came to the definite conclusion that 60 per cent were there as the result of drink."

Accidents, both industrial and other accidents, are commonly the result of the actual incompetence of the worker (or driver of an automobile, etc.) produced by alcohol, or of the carelessness following inhibition of mental control produced by smaller doses of alcohol.

In America for many years past there has been appreciation of the risk of accident in industrial life caused by alcoholic indulgence, and in many directions, as in railway work and in many engineering and other industries, abstinence has been the rule. It has been demonstrated repeatedly that with such abstinence not only is the average output per person at work greatly increased and the loss of days of work greatly reduced, but that also accidents become rarer (see also page 285).

Records of sickness and of mortality display the evil consequences of alcoholic indulgence. I do not propose to give here the comparative experience of groups of total abstainers and of those who take alcohol regularly, though there is no reasonable doubt that even if it be assumed—contrary to the weight of evidence—that abstainers represent a specially selected group, the figures display a smaller amount of sickness and a longer life of abstainers than the general groups, more than is explicable on the hypothesis of selection.

But in group and national experience the contrast as to health and vitality almost necessarily is between abstainers and a mixture of occasional, of moderate, and of excessive drinkers; and as bearing on this, experience in various countries shows the great risks which are incurred through alcoholic indulgence.

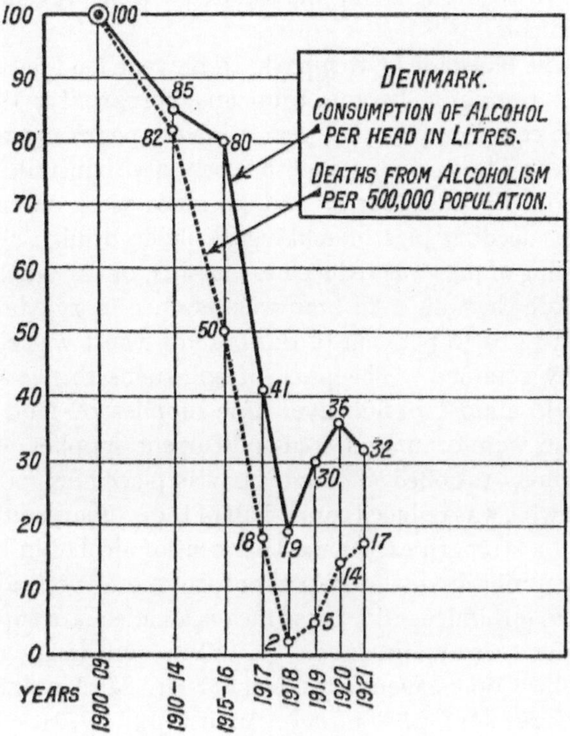


Fig. 10

The experience of England during the Great War demonstrated the value of national and severe restrictions sanctioned and enforced by public opinion as well as by enactments (see page 211, *Health Problems in Organized Society*). The experience of Denmark in the same period, which is summarized in figure 10 brought out the same lesson in preventive medicine.

The blockade of Denmark, to prevent food getting into Germany, became total on February 17, 1917. The cereal crop of that year was very poor; and thus three million people found themselves with insufficient food. At once barley and potatoes were diverted from feeding pigs or making alcoholic drinks. The raising of pigs was reduced to one-fifth of the number before the war. All bran was retained in rye bread and 12 to 15 per cent of the bran of wheat was similarly retained. The price of spirituous drinks was made almost prohibitive. All supplies of food on hand were commandeered and current supplies were severely rationed. A high tax was placed on spirits, brewing was reduced to one-half of the ordinary output and a strength exceeding 3 per cent of alcohol in beer was prohibited. All exports of fruits and vegetables were forbidden. By these means an adequate supply of food was maintained. (A full account is given in "The Copenhagen Experience," Dr. M. Hindhede, *British Medical Journal*, August 12, 1922). The results as regards deaths from alcoholism is shown in figure 10. In this diagram the initial death rate from alcoholism and the initial annual average per capita consumption of alcohol (i.e., for the years 1900–1909) are each stated as 100, while the rates for subsequent groups of years and single years are stated in proportion to this.

The coincidence between the two curves is too striking to find interpretation otherwise than in the altered habits of the community in regard to alcoholic drinks. It is highly improbable that changes in living other than alcoholic had effected the change. Dr. Hindhede gives the further note that prior to the war the death-rate from all causes aged 25 to 65 was 50 to 60 per cent higher in men than in women. This excess he had previously concluded was due to alcohol in men, and not to differences in occupation. During this experimental period the difference between the two sexes had been reduced by about one-half; and would probably have disappeared, had not the female death-rate been also influenced—though to a minor degree by altered alcoholic habits.

Alcoholic consumption has always had a profound influence on family life. Its average economic effect in diverting expenditure from real needs has already been mentioned. At no time is the standard of care and nutrition so important as in the first five years after birth; and in my *Elements of Vital Statistics* and elsewhere I have shown the close relationship between excessive alcoholic consumption and the rate of child mortality. This is due to the lower standard of care, sometimes amounting to actual neglect, produced by alcoholic indulgence. A poorer type of house is occupied than would otherwise be practicable, and thus the risks of infection are multiplied.

Tuberculosis and measles, and many other diseases, are especially prevalent and fatal in the families of the poor; and the risk of invasion of the family by gonorrhea and syphilis is greatly increased by alcoholic indulgence.

The occupational statistics of the English Registrar General demonstrated the risks of handling alcoholic liquors. Thus in 1910–1912, for male adults aged 25 to 65, for a given population the following results are obtained:

| | *Deaths from phthisis* |
|---|---|
| All males | 100 |
| Skilled workmen | 109 |
| Unskilled laborers | 151 |
| Brewers | 127 |
| Publicans | 139 |
| Barmen | 305 |

Not only is disease increased by the lowered resistance to infection produced by alcohol, but also by exposure to excessive doses of infection in saloons and other drinking places.

The history of alcoholic consumption illustrates the evil circles apt to be begun by a single social enemy. Thus in the interrelation of poverty and alcohol: poverty itself increases the temptation to drink, thus intensifying poverty. Poverty means overcrowding, insufficient food, resort to saloons, and usually careless habits, all of which favor tuberculosis, which in its time intensifies and often creates poverty.

The direct and indirect association of alcoholic

consumption with excessive disease is emphasized by its influence on crime and accident. Sullivan has concluded on the basis of experience of British prisons that chronic intoxication is responsible for three-fifths of the homicides, and for many other crimes, including one-fifth of all suicides. Exact observations made by Vernon during the Great War showed that accidents were most numerous in the first shift of work when there were opportunities for getting drink; and that before severe restrictions were introduced and wages were paid on Fridays, accidents were most numerous on Saturdays and Mondays. During the later years 1916–1917 with rigid restrictions on alcohol, accidents were equally distributed through the week. The American National Steel Construction Company had a similar experience. At first three-fourths of the accidents were on Mondays and Tuesdays, after restrictions they were qually distributed each day, and the total not more than half their former number.

As even small doses of alcohol reduce the accuracy and rapidity of action requiring to be taken in response to emergencies, it may well be that during work with complicated machinery or in driving an automobile small doses of alcohol in present conditions of life may be as dangerous as much larger doses in simpler times.

Professor Starling, one of the greatest of modern physiologists, has stated the legitimate limitations of the use of alcohol with an authority which is perhaps even more impressive, because he regarded alcohol as fulfilling a useful function after the end of the day's work, in aiding forgetfulness of the day's troubles and in making man more susceptible "to the operation of the spirit of charity," etc.

As to the food value of alcohol, Starling stated: "the food function is quite unimportant, and is overshadowed by the poisonous action of the drug." Its influence on working capacity is always injurious. As Starling put it:

> For full efficiency alcohol will always have some detrimental effect. A man may do hard work on alcohol, but he will do it in spite of the alcohol and not in virtue of it. . . . . Alcohol should be taken, not before or during work, but when the labors of the day are over, and its main justification will then be not its food value, but the effect which it has on the different functions of the body.

Many experiments have shown that the reflex response to sensory stimuli is definitely retarded by moderate doses of alcohol. This implies retardation of precautionary acts and means increase of the risk of accidents. Other experiments similarly have shown that a moderate dose of alcohol reduces the output of various kinds of work and increases the number of mistakes made.

Starling, alluding to the feelings of well-being produced for instance by a glass of beer, said: "all these results can be ascribed to a paralysing effect of alcohol, which is the first stage of its influence as a narcotic."

McDougall and Smith have grouped alcohol with chloroform, because both raise the resistance of the synapses in all parts of the brain, thus markedly differing from stimulants like tea. Strangely enough this inhibitory influence on work and accuracy of work is associated with a mental impression that the particular task being undertaken after a small dose of alcohol is being performed with unusual quickness and efficiency.

The subject has only been touched on above from a few of its many angles. The outstanding feature of recent years is the practically unanimous conclusion of physicians and of physiologists, that even moderate doses are inimical to good work in life; and we may conclude, that irrespective of the expediency of restrictive measures against alcohol, its dietetic and social use is fraught with serious dangers in personal habit-forming, and in many directions to the rest of the community.

# INDEX OF PROPER NAMES

Abel, J. J., 248

Bacon, Francis, 13
Bacot, 129
Ballard, 98
Bancroft, 136
Banting, 248
Barlow, 269
Bastian, 27
Behring, 64, 68
Bernard, Claude, 19
Block, C. E., 273
Bodington, 189
Bordet, 74, 170
Bryan, 116
Boycott, 123
Bretonneau, 15, 62
Broussais, 16
Brown-Sèquard, 197
Bruce, 107, 141
Buchanan, 91
Buchner, 247
Budd, W., 180
Buhl, 176

Cagniard de la Tour, 24
Carroll, 159
Castiglioni, 152
Carter, H. R., 139, 158, 160
Carter, V., 111
Chamberland, 50, 51
Chauveau, 178
Chick, 264, 269
Cohn, 39
Cohnheim, 177
Cornet, 208
Cramer, 249, 265

Daniels, 149, 151
Darwin, 38
Davy, H., 31
Delepine, 181
Durham, 74

Eberth, 40, 89
Ehrlich, 20, 79, 170, 171
Eijkman, 271
Escherich, 89

Faber, Kund, 15
Farr, 206
Farrell, 124
Findlay, 260
Finlay, 156
Flugge, 197, 207
Funk, 251, 272
Furst, 269

Gaffky, 40
Galen, 175
Gengou, 170
Goethe, 10
Goldberger, 244, 275
Golgi, 145
Gorgas, 156, 157
Grassi, 147, 149
Green, 256
Greenfield, 49

Greenhow, 182, 223
Gull, 234
Guy, W. A., 228

Haffkine, 75
Haldane, J. S., 123, 197, 203
Hartley, H. S., 89, 102
Harvey, 26
Hess, 243, 255, 265
Hill, L., 197, 212, 264
Hindhede, 239, 282
Hippocrates, 13, 175
Holst, 268
Hopkins, J. G., 249, 253, 254, 271
Horrocks, 108
Horsley, 234
Hrdlicka, 166
Huldschinsky, 215, 265
Hunter, J., 168
Hutchinson, J., 167
Huxley, 10, 26, 34

Jenner, 72

Kemball, 237
Kitasato, 75, 128
Klebs, 42
Koch, 35, 39, 86, 171, 178, 185, 214
Kocher, 234

Laennec, 15, 176
Laveran, 145, 170
Lavoisier, 196
Lazear, 159
Leeuenhoeck, 24
Lewis, 136
Liebreich, 19
Lister, 31
Loeffler, 40
Loeb, 5
Long, W., 59
Looss, 121
Lunin, 249

MacCallum, 139, 147
Manson, 134, 135, 146
Marine, 233
Maxcy, 113
McCollum, 231, 252, 254, 261
McGarrison, 236, 244
McKnee, 117
Mellanby, 215, 253, 256, 262
Mendel, 244
Metschnikoff, 73, 169
Norton, 31, 175
Myers, 229

Nageli, 203
Nicolle, 112
Niemeyer, 176
Niven, J., 135
Nocard, 54
Noguchi, 169
Nott, J., 156
Nuttall, 73, 135

Obermeier, 111
Ord, W. M., 234
Osborne, 244

Paget, 29, 58
Park, 69, 101
Pasteur, 19, 21, 23, 46, 52
Pettenkofer, 83, 196

Pfeiffer, 51, 74
Power, W. H., 98
Pringle, 206

Ramazzini, 220
Ransome, 181, 188
Redi, 25
Reed, W., 156, 158
Ricketts, 113
Rosenheim, 263
Rosenau, 143
Ross, R., 145, 146
Roux, 48, 50, 55, 63, 169

Sanderson, B., 177
Schafer, 233
Schaudinn, 169
Schick, 68, 77
Sedgwick, 96
Semmelweiss, 35
Simon, J., 84
Simond, 129
Simpson, 30
Smith, Theobald, 77, 134, 138, 186
Snow, J., 83
Spallanzani, 26
Starling, 247, 285
Stiles, 124
Still, J. F., 270
Sydenham, 20
Sylvius, 175

Thackrah, 14, 221, 238
Thompson, A., 129
Thorne, 114
Trousseau, 18
Trudeau, 189
Turner, G., 105
Tyndall, 27, 207

Vernon, 198, 285
Villemin, 18, 177
Virchow, 17, 176

Wassermann, 75, 169
Weigert, 42
Wells, 31
Widal, 74
Winslow, 97
Woodhead, 97
Wright, 73, 75

Yersin, 63, 128

Zingher, 69

# INDEX OF SUBJECTS

(See also Contents, pages vii–xii)


Accessory food factors, 250
Accidents and alcohol, 280
Age and deaths, 9
Air and ventilation, 195
Alcoholism, 227, 277
Anaesthetics, 19, 31
Anopheles, 146
Ankylostomiasis, 120
Anthrax, 41, 225
Antitoxin, 64
Anti-typhoid inoculation, 76
Attenuation of virulence, 48, 55
Arsenical treatment, 170

Bacteriological technique, 39
Beri-beri, 270
Biogenesis, 26
Bread, 244
Brill's disease, 113

Calomel in prophylaxis, 169
Carbon monoxide, 199
Carriers, 87, 100
Cancer, 226
Causes of death, 7
Causation, 12, 22
Cellular pathology, 18
Chemo-therapeutics, 79
Chicken cholera, 47
Chlorination of water, 98
Cholera, 75, 81
Cleanliness, 114
Cod liver oil, 244, 259, 264
Cretinism, 233

Deficiency diseases, 259
Dietaries, 242
Diphtheria, 60
Dosage of infection, 185
Ductless glands, 21
Dust and disease, 222

Elephantiasis, 136
Enteric fever, 16, 77, 87, 88
Epidemic constitution, 12, 67
Epidemicity, 67, 70, 158
Ergosterol, 263

Fatigue, 228
Fermentation, 24, 37, 247
"Fever" hospitals, 114
Filariasis, 134
Filter-passing virus, 163
Filtration of water, 86, 96
Flachery, 38
Fleas and plague, 129
Flies and disease, 134
Fog, 211
Food deficiencies, 241

Gluttony, 14, 238
Goats and infection, 108
Goitre, 233
Gonorrhoea, 164
Gout, 239

Helio-therapy, 216
Hookworm disease, 120
Hormones, 246
Hospitals, 29, 206
Housing, 207, 217

Immunity, 64, 69, 72, 79, 188
Industrial occupations, 207, 220
Inebriety, 279
Inoculation, disease by, 54, 159, 169
Insect-borne disease, 156
Iodine treatment, 236

Keratomalacia, 273

Lead poisoning, 224
Lemon juice, 255
Liver fats, 252, 256
Louse-borne disease, 111

Malaria, 20, 143
Malnutrition, 185, 240
Marsh miasm, 144
Malta fever, 106
Mexican typhus, 113
Midwifery, 35
Milk, 244, 254, 263
Milk infection, 98
Miner's anaemia, 123
Mosquito, 137, 156
Muzzling of dogs, 58
Myxoedema, 235

Occupation, 183, 217, 220
Ontology, 17, 20
Operations, 35
Organic effluvia, 197
Ovariotomy, 30
Oysters, 98

Pandemics, 132
Pellagra, 274
Pébrine, 37
Pfeiffer's phenomenon, 74
Phagocytosis, 73
Phthisis, 175, 223
Physiological medicine, 17
Plague, 77, 126
Plasmodium, 145
Phosphorus fumes, 224
Poverty, 183
Prophylaxis, 47
Protozoa and disease, 141, 169
Purification of water, 95
Putrefaction, 33

Quarantine, 87
Quinine, 20, 152

Rabies, 52
Rat plague, 128
Relapsing fever, 111
Rickets, 257

Salvarsan, 20, 80, 170
Sanitary defects, 104, 124, 201
Scarlet fever, 78
Scurvy, 254, 267
Secretin, 247
Serological tests, 74, 107, 170
Shell-fish, 87, 98
Sleeping sickness, 171
Smoke, 211
Specificity, 15
Spirochaete, 169

Spontaneous generation, 25
Sterilization, 28
Syphilis, 20, 80, 164
Suctorial insects, 146
Sunlight, 211, 262, 265
Sunlight and infection, 181
Stegomyia, 159

Texas fever, 135, 138
Treatment for prevention, 125, 172, 188, 236
Technique, 43
Terrain and microbe, 179
Tetanus, 75
Ticks, 140
Toxin-antitoxin, 69
Trench fever, 116
Trypanosomes, 142, 170
Tuberculisation, 187
Tuberculosis, 15, 18, 174
Typhus fever, 112, 115

Ultra-violet rays, 215, 263, 265
Undulant fever, 106
Urbanization, 218

Vaccination, 48, 58, 89
Variability of bacteria, 40, 88
Venereal diseases, 164
Ventilation, 195
Vitamins, 246

Water supplies, 84, 90
Widal reaction, 74

Yellow fever, 154